MW00594302

LIFE
Reimagined

WOMEN'S STORIES OF HOPE, RESILIENCE & TRANSFORMATION

Compiled by Linda Joy
Edited by Deborah Kevin

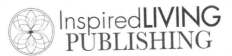

InspiredLIVING
PUBLISHING

Life Reimagined
Copyright © Linda Joy 2021

All rights reserved. No part of this publication may be reproduced, stored in a retrieval system, or transmitted in any form or by any means, electronic, mechanical, photocopying, recording, scanning, or otherwise, except as permitted under Section 107 or 108 of the 1976 United States Copyright Act, without the prior written permission of the publisher. Requests to publisher for permission should be addressed to the Permissions Department, Inspired Living Publishing, P.O. Box 1149, Lakeville, MA 02347 or by e-mail at Linda@ InspiredLivingPublishing.com.

Limit of Liability/Disclaimer of Warranty. The Publisher makes no representation or warranties with respect to the accuracy or completeness of the contents of this work and specifically disclaims all warranties, including without limitation warranties of fitness for a particular purpose. No warranty may be created or extended by sales or promotional materials. The advice and strategies contained herein may not be suitable for every situation. This work is sold with the understanding that the Publisher is not engaged in rendering legal, accounting, counseling, or other professional services. If such assistance is required, the services of a competent professional should be sought. Neither the Publisher nor the Editor shall be liable for damages arising therefrom. The fact that an Author's organization or website is referred to in this work as a potential source of further information does not mean that the Publisher endorses the information the organization or website may provide, or recommendations it may make.

Trade paperback ISBN: 978-1-7327425-4-3
eBook ISBN: 978-1-7327425-5-0
Library of Congress Control Number: 2021947788

Published by Inspired Living Publishing, LLC.
P.O. Box 1149, Lakeville, MA 02347
InspiredLivingPublishing.com
(508) 265-7929

Cover Design: Mandy Gates www.GruveDesign.com
Interior Design & Layout: Patricia Creedon www.patcreedondesign.com
Editor: Deborah Kevin, www.DeborahKevin.com
Linda Joy Photo Credit: Ali Rosa Photography www.alirosaphotography.com

Printed in the United States.

Dedication

This book is dedicated to...

Every woman who has had to dig deep to find the courage to step beyond her perceived limitations and into the unknown. You are stronger than you know and braver than you can imagine.

Every woman who, in honoring the calling of the still, small voice within, has taken her first steps on the winding path to authenticity.

Every woman who bravely chooses to brush aside fear and self-doubt, and peel back the layers that hide or dim her divine light.

Every woman who reaches with an outstretched hand to uplift, empower, and support other women in living a technicolor life.

And, also to...

Niki, my beautiful daughter: you inspire me with your wide-open heart, loving compassion, and beautiful soul. I am honored beyond words that you were gifted to me in this lifetime. Watching you with your daughter is one of the greatest blessings of my life.

Makenna (aka "The Little Goddess"), my spirited, creative, love-filled nine-year-old granddaughter: you took my heart by storm and reminded me that joy and happiness are within reach when we allow ourselves to be fully in the moment. May you always embrace your magic and magnificence, my love, and never dull your sparkle.

Tyler, my grandson: you inspire me with your loving, compassionate heart and your quest to find balance and fairness in the world around you. May you remember your truth and magic and find the greatest peace and happiness in that truth.

Dana, my soul mate, best friend, love of my life: twenty-seven years in, you still make my heart skip a beat, bring a smile to my lips, and make me feel like the most important woman in the world. I'm truly blessed.

The multitude of extraordinary women who have come into my life over the last thirty years of my spiritual journey. Whether for a moment or a lifetime, your brilliant spirits and open hearts have touched and inspired me beyond words. My greatest wish is that I might light the way for others as you have for me.

To the authors of *Life Reimagined* who have trusted me to share their sacred soul stories with the world. Your bravery through the sometimes-painful writing process continues to inspire me.

The extraordinary team of talented women with whom I have been honored, blessed, and humbled to work with to bring this project to life: Deborah Kevin, editor on this sacred project, who brings the essence of each story to light; Patricia Creedon for the beautiful interior design, Mandy Gates for the stunning cover design, and Kim Turcotte, my Goddess of Operations and soul sister, who, for over a decade, organizes and brings my visions to life.

And finally, to ...

You, the reader—the beautiful, deserving recipient of the love and light in these pages. I am grateful our paths crossed at this moment and time. May you always. May you live your life in technicolor—filled with unbridled passion, truth, and joy.

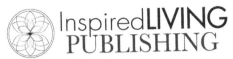

InspiredLIVING PUBLISHING

www.InspiredLivingPublishing.com

Inspired Living Publishing's bestselling titles include:

The Art of Self-Nurturing: A Field Guide to Living with More Peace, Joy & Meaning by Kelley Grimes, MSW

Broken Open: Embracing Heartache and Betrayal as Gateways to Unconditional Love by Mal Duane

Soul-Hearted Living: A Year of Sacred Reflections & Affirmations for Women by Dr. Debra Reble

Everything Is Going to Be Okay! From the Projects to Harvard to Freedom by Dr. Catherine Hayes, CPCC

Being Love: How Loving Yourself Creates Ripples of Transformation in Your Relationship and the World by Dr. Debra Reble

Awakening to Life: Your Sacred Guide to Consciously Creating a Life of Purpose, Magic, and Miracles by Patricia Young

The Art of Inspiration: An Editor's Guide to Writing Powerful, Effective Inspirational & Personal Development Books by Bryna Haynes

As well as these bestselling titles in ILP's sacred anthology division:

SHINE! Stories to Inspire You to Dream Big, Fear Less & Blaze Your Own Trail

Courageous Hearts: Soul-Nourishing Stories to Inspire You to Embrace Your Fears and Follow Your Dreams

Midlife Transformation: Redefining Life, Love, Health and Success

Inspiration for a Woman's Soul: Opening to Gratitude & Grace

Inspiration for a Woman's Soul: Cultivating Joy

Inspiration for a Woman's Soul: Choosing Happiness

Embracing Your Authentic Self: Women's Stories of Self-Discovery & Transformation

Juicy, Joyful Life: Inspiration from Women Who Have Found the Sweetness in Every Day

Unleash Your Inner Magnificence (ebook only)

The Wisdom of Midlife Women 2 (ebook only)

You can find the majority of the titles at major online retailers and at bookstores by request.

LIFE *Reimagined*

PRAISE FOR
Life Reimagined

"Vulnerable. Empowering. Filled with Hope. *Life Reimagined* features twenty transformational stories by women that will inspire you to believe in possibility, hold on to hope, and to release the weight of self-doubt."

–**Amy Leigh Mercree**, bestselling author of fifteen books including *100 Days to Calm*

"*Life Reimagined* is full of touching and inspiring stories of ways these authors reimagined their dreams, self, relationships, and spirit. The reflection questions will guide you to discover more of your own soul wisdom. Enjoy."

– **Lisa Michaels**, speaker, author, and CEO Impact Certifications

"*Life Reimagined* is a moving collection of inspirational stories from women who said *yes* to honoring their truth and living their best lives. This empowering book inspires women to listen to their inner guides and to begin living their life in full color! The reflective journal prompts at the end of each story invite you to dive deeper into your own story."

– **Dr. Margaret Paul**, bestselling author/co-author of *Do I Have to Give Up Me to Be Loved by You? Inner Bonding, Healing Your Aloneness, Diet for Divine Connection,* and *The Inner Bonding Workbook*

"*Life Reimagined* gives the reader an up-close look at the unstoppable strength, courage, and resilience of women. These truth tellers share moments of profound transformation and a split second of divine revelation. Each writer takes you down a pathway of awakening to an inner voice and seeing the uncovering of their soul's desires. Each story ignites a spark of inspiration in the reader."

– **Mal Duane**, crystal master, emotional healer and bestselling author

"*Life Reimagined* is poignant and soul-stirring. An absolute must-read for women in the throes of reinvention. Discover deeply touching stories of courage, creativity, and perseverance in the face of life-altering transformation. Each story offers life lessons every woman can relate to and learn from. You will come away inspired!"

– **Shann Vander Leek**, award-winning producer and podcast coach

"*Life Reimagined* takes us into the heart of women's stories of transformation from the inside out. I love the reflective questions at the end of each story! These inquiries are like portals for great self-discovery for readers. A deep calling forth to live our best lives is invited and inspired within the pages of this book."

– **Lynda Monk**, director, International Association for Journal Writing

"See yourself and your own personal growth journey in these true, inspiring, transformational stories of women who have survived and thrived after every kind of trauma imaginable."

– **Arielle Ford**, author and love coach

"Witnessing a woman bravely transform her life, whether by choice or circumstance, is powerful. That is the essence of the deeply personal stories shared in this inspiring book. Each story adeptly illustrates that, even in the darkest times, there is a way to happiness if you trust and reimagine what's possible."

– **Kelly Mishell**, mindset coach, speaker, and bestselling author

"Dreams really do come true! Linda Joy and her beautiful circle of authors have done it again. This book is full of inspiring true stories that made me laugh, made me cry, and, most of all, made me have hope for myself and for the world. The deep and honest sharing of these women's personal stories is poignant, and I see myself reflected in many of the journeys shared here. Whether you dip into a story here and there or read it cover to cover, you will be delighted by what you find in *Life Reimagined*."

— **Minette Riordan, Ph.D.**, creativity coach, artist, and author

"Pure inspiration! What a beautiful creation! Each woman's story made me feel like I was sitting in her living room, sipping tea, and listening to her story. This book gives me faith in the power of women and the transformation that can happen when we choose positive change over fear. Love rules!"

— **Elvia Roe,** angel alchemist and expert teacher at AngelsTeach.com

"I am moved and marveled by the miraculous collection of transformational stories in this beautiful book. These brave women all share a sacred piece of their heart as they unwind their deeply personal journey's through a seemingly impossible problem out the other end to a realization of the gift within each conflict. After reading this, you will discover your own courage to reimagine your life changing in ways you only once dreamed of."

— **Carrie Rowan,** international bestselling author of *Tell A New Story*, mindset and energy coach, and professor of empowerment and joy

"*Life Reimagined* is a powerful book sharing not just stories, but the hearts and souls of women from different lives, different backgrounds, and challenges, who emerge stronger and more in touch with who they truly are. Despite what these women separately endured, they learned through their own journey, to overcome self-doubt, fear, and much more to truly find, embrace, and reimagine a spiritual home within themselves. In turn, they offer us faith, hope, and the knowledge that we too can discover or rediscover that place within ourselves that vibrates with personal strength to live our best lives closely connected to our spiritual truth and essence."

—**Dr. Jo Anne White**, international, #1 bestselling, award-winning author, certified professional coach, consultant, and energy master teacher

Foreword

CHRISTY WHITMAN

When my friend and colleague, Linda Joy, who I've known since the early 2000s, asked me to write the foreword for this book, I was deeply honored because Linda is a shining example of a woman who is clear about her passion and dedicated to do whatever it takes to remain in alignment with that purpose. And, like Linda and the rest of the remarkable women whose stories you'll read on these pages, I too have reimagined and recreated my life—not once but many times, both personally and professionally.

I've lived through a divorce, my sister's suicide, and the open-heart surgery and month-long hospitalization that saved the life of my newborn son. Before I came to understand that life is not something that happens *to* us, but something that unfolds *from* us and *for* us, I felt like a victim of just about everything and everyone around me. Life felt like an uphill battle, and no matter how hard I worked, I wasn't gaining any ground.

Back then, I was thirty pounds overweight and more than $60,000 in debt. I worked at a job I hated and had a knack for attracting the "wrong" kind of men. And despite having achieved all the outer symbols of career success, I was deeply unfulfilled and unhappy, even while knowing in my heart that there had to be something more.

Like the women whose stories of hope, resilience, and transformation form the basis of this book, I have also learned some important lessons and universal principles that continue to guide me back to my power and have supported me in creating an abundant, empowered life that would have been virtually unrecognizable to the woman I was in my twenties. And something I know with certainty now that I didn't know then is that contrasting or painful life experiences always come bearing invaluable gifts. They show us where we've fallen out of alignment with the Divine energy stream that sources us, so we can make our way back to our own inner truth and allow a purer, higher frequency to guide our choices. Contrast makes us aware of the bigger life that is calling us, while simultaneously showing us where we are still settling for less and playing small.

There are only two fundamental attitudes we can hold in relation to any important aspect of our lives. We can relate to ourselves as being powerless over the circumstances that surround us, or we can accept ourselves as powerful creators who can at any moment shift our perspective and change our trajectory. And when we begin to actively look for the ways that each relationship and situation is serving us, we discover that everything truly is.

The turning points in our lives that we relish and adore—those moments when we can feel the wind begin to change and the fulcrum start to tip in our favor...when we see the first glimmer of hope that an unwanted situation has the potential of improving—these turning points are the natural consequence of making an inner shift in our own energy fields that is felt and answered by everything and everyone around us. For as vibrational beings who are both energy transmitters and energy receivers, everything we draw into our lives is in direct response to the vibration we send out. We are alchemists with the power to spin straw into gold, and it is every woman's very personal and spiritual journey to reawaken to this power within her.

The real-life stories shared here will do much more than entertain or inspire you; they'll reawaken you to the importance of heeding your intuition and will help you recognize the presence of your Divine source that is always guiding you. And though each woman you'll meet has transcended her own unique set of circumstances, all of them have discovered a common truth: There is tremendous power in alignment. When we're in a state of vibrational alignment within the private inner world of our hearts and minds, doors in the outer world magically open, and things we once viewed as problems or even tragedies reveal themselves as blessings in disguise.

For thousands of years, women have come together to share their stories and their struggles, to immerse ourselves in our rich inner worlds and renew ourselves with the energy of the Divine feminine. This book will support you in stepping back from the demands of your daily life to drink from the collective wisdom of this extraordinary circle of women. I invite you to allow their courage to recharge and inspire you, and to take the clues they offer for how to listen with greater attention when your intuition begins nudging you in a new direction.

Whatever challenges you may currently be facing—whether you're struggling with early-life trauma, personal loss, career uncertainty, unhealthy patterns in your relationships with others, or simply navigating one of the many natural times of transition in every woman's life—you will find within these pages hard-won wisdom and valuable insights to help you find your way back to your creative power and stand in a new possibility for your life.

Christy Whitman
Channel for The Quantum Council
ChristyWhitman.com

TABLE OF
Contents

LIFE

Reimagined

WOMEN'S STORIES OF HOPE, RESILIENCE & TRANSFORMATION

Introduction

LINDA JOY

As a high-school drop-out, former welfare mom, and queen of self-sabotage, I know first-hand the power of reimagining one's life through a lens of possibility instead of the *shoulds, have tos*, expectations of others, and the negative narrative that so often runs in the background.

It's been thirty years since those days, and I still clearly remember the evenings spent curled up next to my then seven-year-old daughter, envisioning the life I wanted for myself, for her, and for my soul—a life filled with love, joy, fulfillment, and peace. I'd envision the details in full technicolor with all of my emotions and senses engaged. What I thought at the time might be just a 'magical escape' was really my soul showing me what was possible.

Today, I am living the life I imagined.

In October 2020, during a time of personal challenge, deep reflection, and a global pandemic, the title of *Life Reimagined* dropped into my awareness as I sat in an overstuffed chair in a Boston hotel room staring out the window at the wing of Massachusetts General Hospital sending focused healing energy to the love of my life, Dana, as he underwent delicate surgery for a large brain aneurysm. It was his second major surgery since we'd learned in November 2019 of his dual diagnosis of a pituitary tumor and an aneurysm.

At that moment, my soul knew *Life Reimagined* would be the next book in Inspired Living Publishing's sacred anthology series. I knew there were other women who, even before the global pandemic, had reimagined their lives one or more times, and I felt it was crucial to share those stories.

As I sat there, with my hand on my heart, sending protective energy to Dana and prayers of divine support for his surgical team, I was filled with this sense of deep inner peace that I had never experienced at the depth before—and a knowing—a deep soul knowing—that *no matter what* happened in that surgical room over the next two hours—I wouldn't be the same. Instead, I would move forward with a deeper commitment to living the intentional life Dana and I had created as well as a more profound commitment to supporting women in doing the same.

It was in that moment of deep reflection that the title of this book dropped in, and the vision for the cover came through, showing a burst of light coming from the darkness.

An hour later, I received the call I knew would come: all was well post-surgery, and Dana was thriving.

Each of the twenty powerful women in this book has experienced her midlife wake-up call, whether the message was delivered through a personal night of the soul, a health scare, a relationship crisis, a career meltdown, or a dream reignited, its message rang through loud and clear, "Life isn't meant to be lived in black and white, devoid of love, radiant health, fulfilling relationships, success, and self-worth. Simply existing. Life is meant to be lived in technicolor, filled with unbridled passion, truth, and joy."

It takes a great deal of courage, grit, and perseverance to change course in the middle of your life, and the women who have contributed to this book embody all three.

For some women, their transformations required monumental shifts in the physical realm; for others, change unfolded from within like a blooming lotus and gently peeled away the layers of fear, expectation, and conditioning that kept them stuck in a life that no longer fit.

In these transformational stories, you'll see many manifestations of courage, hope, and resilience. All of them will inspire you. Some of them may echo your own story and, perhaps, you'll recognize the whispers of your own soul on these pages.

Beautiful soul, allow these stories to remind you of the truth that you are strong enough to choose a new path, resilient enough to overcome whatever challenges come your way, and that you deserve the life, love, and happiness that you envision.

May this book be a supportive guide along your way.

Live an Intentional & Inspired Life,

Linda Joy
Bestselling Publisher

CHAPTER ONE

DREAMS
Reimagined

From Answering the Phone to Starring in My Own Life

JAMI HEARN

*O*nce a month, for nearly a year, I had been sneaking out of work early. I arrived by 6 a.m. that day, so no one could say I hadn't billed enough hours. I excitedly strode across the parking lot and took the steps to my office two at a time. I almost didn't even notice the hideous striped wallpaper surrounding the windowless box where I spent the majority of my waking hours. The excitement of my destination after work made up, mostly, for the fluorescent lights that would be searing my senses for the next eleven plus hours.

By the end of what seemed like the longest day ever, I decreed that all of the chaos and disorder that covered my desk would still be there the next morning. I closed the file I'd been working on, locked my door, changed out of my straight-jacket-like suit and claimed my freedom for the night.

My car was a portal. For the next hour, I soaked in blaring rock and roll with the windows down, letting the wave of freedom wash over me. I arrived for dinner with my normal gang in a completely refreshed mental state. My companions were not just ordinary dinner-goers. These were my psychic-medium and shaman friends. I felt their frequency before I was even out of my car.

Inside the restaurant, we discussed the show that was about to air, the energies swirling and the spirits surrounding us that evening. I was the guest host for my friend's television show, she did call-in psychic readings. Occasionally, for the studio audience, she would tap into the guides, teachers, and loved ones that were present.

I was inspired and in awe of this demonstration of connection. She was a fountain of information and messages from the realm that was beyond vision for so many. I existed on the cusp of this space. I had always been connected to spirit and had spent most of my adult life ignoring it. I felt the pull to allow this part of me to peek through the curtain. I had been hiding behind the cape of my own fears and doubts. I was ready to open that cape, just a bit.

In that studio, with a deck of folded, stained tarot cards, three crystals, and two feathers, I answered the phone and welcomed callers to the special hour of messages. The vibration of those messages and the women I shared that room with, left me unable to sleep for days. I knew a part of me was awakening. An unfamiliar, unseen part that seemed to fill all the gaps began emerging. Once the bottle opened, there was no putting the Genie back. This was the true me and it felt exactly right…at least inside that bubble, I rode the wave of excitement that I hadn't felt since I was a child.

The next day, trying to focus on the mire of work in front of me felt like moving through quicksand, with images of the fun and connection sprinkled in from the night before. Everyone around me went on about their mindless toiling, just like every other Thursday, waiting for lunch to come, gossiping around the water cooler, and surfing on the Internet, pretending to bill hours for the firm. There was no one in my everyday life that had any inkling of what was happening behind my cape. I was feeling more alone than I ever had, hiding behind the cape I wore for security, so no one could see me.

How could two completely different versions of me be existing in the same human body? The night before, I was brimming with excitement, anticipation, and joy. And, now I felt adrift, no oar, bumping into buoys, being steered by a machine where I was nothing but a cog. I found myself longing to allow the spiritual, excited, connected part of me to emerge. The longer I stuffed it down and pretended it wasn't there, the more resentment I began to harbor. It was time to honor my truth.

I started noticing unusual things around me. Like the night Joan of Arc sat on the edge of my bed to support me through depression as my marriage was ending, and I felt like I couldn't find which end was up. Or the auras I saw around pregnant women, sometimes before they even knew they were expecting. Turns out these new experiences were becoming a normal part of the me that I was beginning to acknowledge. I could no longer just pretend my intuition wasn't screaming and my cape wasn't peeling itself back. And of course, unsolicited fun facts would pop out of my mouth without much management. Like the time I saw a client and before he spoke, I asked who was representing his wife. He stammered in response that he hadn't even told me his wife left him. The time had come to get a handle on my new insights!

I was beginning to see the integration of spirit with who I was in the outside world. The disconnection between who I pretended to be and forced myself to show up as, was also glaringly apparent. The harder I pressed myself to conform to the expectations of others, the more reticent I became. Every challenge that led me to continue denying who I was at soul level, also led me to feel more and more anger rising up within me.

Finally, I was presented with the opportunity I had been secretly longing for. A friend was hosting a psychic fair, and I quietly yearned to participate, but wasn't brave and confident enough to reserve a spot. I happened to cross paths with this friend. I believe she was the messenger sent to kick my ass into motion, even though I had no vision of the roller coaster I was about to embark on. She asked what I was doing that Saturday, to which I responded that I wasn't sure yet.

"Great, be ready at 7:30, set-up has to be complete by 9:00—see you then!" She hadn't given me the opportunity to second guess myself. I had less than forty-eight hours to organize my first professional reading appearance. I barely even uttered the word psychic, let alone held myself out to be one. This was the real test to see if I could leave my cape of security and invisibility at home.

That morning, I arrived, and set up my table in a space that was chaotic and noisy. But I was a pro at navigating circumstances like those. I settled in and allowed myself to relax into a space of connection with my true self, with my soul. There I had no pretenses, no reservations. I reveled in the truest expression of who I was.

That weekend I delivered wisdom and guidance to more than twenty souls. I could barely speak by the end of the event. I felt so grateful to my friend for pushing me to show up and for bringing me snacks throughout the day. This gave me a glimpse into parts of me that had been hidden behind my cape, some I hadn't been willing to look at previously.

I took that springboard as the pivot point to curate my experience; to live, daily, inside that vibration and frequency where I operated fully uncloaked and visible. I released the shackles of expectation from the outside world and leapt into the pool of pure bliss that allowed me to get really comfortable with who I was at soul level. I also got the privilege of navigating the world of spirit where my clients and I sought guidance, healing, and insights.

I unlocked access to the truest version of me and I now share it with the world. I am no longer concerned with the expectations (or billable hours) of my former life. Perhaps the best part of this life I have built from images in my imagination is seeing how my brazen approach to who I am and my spiritual connection impacts all those I meet. I even get to witness the ripple impact. It's not always immediate, but my birth into the most authentic expression of myself wasn't all that quick either. I had lots of convincing to do, as I claimed my sovereignty.

This is real freedom; being embodied in who I truly am, every damn day!

Reflection

Is there a part of who you are that you haven't been able to look at? What if you could? What's the best that could happen? What's the worst?

_____

_____

_____

_____

How do you define and embody your personal freedom? Where are you allowing the expectations of others to infringe on your sovereignty?

_____

_____

_____

_____

Where have you gotten little peeks at the true version of you that is ready to shine through? If you aren't leaning into that version of you, what is holding you back?

_____

_____

_____

_____

Spiritual Sovereignty: Hindsight is 20/20

LISA MANYON

*W*hen 2020 began, I felt like I was on top of the world. I had retained many fabulous clients, doing the work that I love. My Healing With Love journey was gaining traction. I was invited to do an author reading and signing for the #1 International Bestseller *The Silver Lining of Cancer*, at our local bookstore. I was in my element, surrounded by books and community, at one of the most amazing Q & A sessions I've ever experienced. Books were sold and signed. Deep connections were made. The impact of my healing story was evident, as people were asking me how I managed to become cancer-free without chemo or radiation. The miracle of experiencing cancer had become a catalyst for helping humanity to heal, by demonstrating how we can reclaim our health, amplify our vibration, lean into faith, and create our reality.

Several years prior, on May 16, 2017, I heard three words that would change the trajectory of my life. "You have cancer." OR maybe it was, "It is cancer." Either way, as my ENT delivered the news to my mom and me, I sat there soaking it in, breathing through it, and embracing what was next. I felt some disbelief and some relief... I knew it was time to heal with love. This deep knowing came from the divinely guided message, "*you will heal with love*" that I received prior to diagnosis. That felt way better than the alternative. I surrendered into a peaceful calm, while I prepared myself to follow the threads and heal, with love, or gracefully make my exit. That night, I sipped on the prosecco I had purchased to celebrate "good news" and had a deep cleansing cry.

What followed was a complete lifestyle reset on all levels. Facing mortality was the moment I reimagined my life. Fast forward to 2020; after two major surgeries, lots of love, and intensive healing work with multiple traditional and alternative practitioners—I was cancer-free and sharing my story to inspire others.

And then, the world stopped. At least the world as we'd known it. The pandemic was in full swing, and businesses shut down. We were told to stay home and only leave for necessities. Humanity panicked, masks became mandatory, and the great divide deepened in historic pandemic fashion. Devastating wildfires in Southern Oregon, and long overdue cultural shifts, led to unrest on many levels. I call this time the perpetual unknown or unknowing. Because of the great divide between political parties, vaxxers, and anti-vaxxers, media censorship, racism, and more, truth became lies, and lies became truth.

I decided, in a moment of deep meditation, that if the world was going to end, I was going to swim. I journaled about my ideal space in a housing market with less than a two percent vacancy rate. Within two weeks I manifested what I desired, a beautiful home complete with swimming pool, large kitchen, primary en suite bedroom with walk-in closet, office space, guest room, and a yard with rose bushes. Interestingly, the space had sat vacant for four months as if it were waiting for me. I took this as a good sign and reveled in the vibration of my new digs. Despite this pocket of joy in my life, the world seemingly continued to spin out of control.

I lost three important people: my uncle, kindergarten teacher, and a life-long friend (none were COVID-19 related, but were devastating losses nonetheless). World health dictated social distancing, and hugs became acts of rebellion. Depression was on the rise, including my own. On multiple levels, I simultaneously experienced heartbreak and heart-opening. I felt as though I had lost my magic. I experienced my first and only bout of TMJ, necessitating physical therapy to loosen my jaw. I could barely open my mouth (another form of trying to suppress my voice and not fully being valued, heard, or seen, perhaps).

It was everything I could do to maintain my sanity, peace of mind, and faith. My stress levels were high, and this is especially concerning for me. As a cancer thriver, I know the importance of energetic integrity and taking care of the body, mind, and spirit. All are paramount to BEing healthy and at peace. For the most part, I stayed in my little bubble. Despite the slight sense of security gained by tapping into conveniences like InstaCart grocery delivery, I felt the collective fear permeating my sacred sphere of influence. As a highly intuitive empath, it takes extra effort for me to manage my energy and not take on the weight of the world.

In times of unrest, when collective fear permeates the atmosphere, the perpetual unknowing hangs thick in the air, showering us with doubt and sucking the hope and joy from our hearts. It is too easy to give our voice and power away, without even realizing it. When seeking, we often turn to gurus, healers, teachers, coaches, mentors, and even well-meaning friends who don't hold the key to our inner truth. I did everything I could to maintain my energetic integrity, including deep healing work with some trusted and not so trusted healers. I learned difficult lessons about allowing others into my energy field. These lessons rolled over into 2021 and my sacred sphere of influence.

I navigated these life-altering experiences seeking support from healers and light-workers, some of whom were Spiritual Groomers and Spiritual Charlatans/Shysters. I was clearly shown how many healers manipulate the vulnerability of others for their gain. I experienced breaches of trust, and boundaries were crossed. One healer attempted to play a fatherly role in my life, began to gain trust, and started pushing additional sessions when they were not necessary. My struggle with depression was shared, without permission, by a trusted friend to a partner practitioner, who did not have my best interest at heart. This person tried to sabotage my work, and my health, and project on to me that "almost all people suffering from depression are not living their purpose." This person systematically drove a wedge between my previously trusted friend and me, in the guise of "love and light."

What I discovered is that the truth of those healers was not my truth. I was shown how they were trying to manipulate others. I realized that things get wonky when I become separated from my direct connection with my higher self and God. Thankfully I came full circle back to my faith. But, not before experiencing powerful lessons, including the importance of energetic integrity and the damage energetic interference can cause.

Not all things are as they seem, and many times stories are conjured, influenced, and shaped by half-truths that have been projected to impact your worldview. Spiritual Charlatans/Shysters and Spiritual Groomers are often self-proclaimed healers who promote themselves as trusted advisers and share many of the same patterns. They lack boundaries, exhibit unhealthy dark undertones and deep personal agendas both consciously and subconsciously. They are masters of cloaking their true essence shrouded in the guise of "love and light" while imparting great harm on those they claim to serve.

It's now clear to me that when organizations, and "healers", and their interests, and beliefs begin to stealthily infiltrate my sacred space, trying to influence me in manipulative ways, it's time to take a step back. When experiencing people and situations like this, I've learned to question everything, break the trance, challenge the status quo, and engage in critical thinking.

By Being fully aligned with my truth, intuition, faith, and direct connection with Source (God, the Universe, Creator, Gaia, or whatever term resonates), the veil was lifted, and it all became crystal clear and certain. I simultaneously regained my energetic integrity and Spiritual Sovereignty, I reclaimed my essence, and I can feel the magic of life again. I gave myself grace when releasing people, places, and things that no longer serve. I learned to let go and allow the journey to unfold for others without my input or influence.

What I wish for YOU today is Spiritual Sovereignty. May you hold fast to your ability to connect with your higher self directly through the Creator. May you embrace only pure love. May you break through the illusions of guruism, losing your voice and giving your power away.

Do not let others influence or derail your purpose. Trust your faith. It is your direct connection with Source that leads to Spiritual Sovereignty. This is when you know you've come home to yourself and have finally tapped into Spiritual Sugar, the inner sweetness of your soul where you can heal yourself with love.

Reflection

Where are you giving your power and your voice away?

_____

_____

_____

_____

How can you trust your intuition more?

_____

_____

_____

_____

In what ways are you deepening your faith to strengthen your Spiritual Sovereignty?

_____

_____

_____

_____

Hawaiian Dreams

DR. LISA THOMPSON

*O*ne evening in May 2020, I was having dinner with my husband and daughter at our home in Olympia, Washington. We had been stuck in lockdown due to COVID-19 for two months, with no indication of when things would get better.

My daughter, out of the blue, said, "I want to move to Malibu, California, to surf."

Without thinking, I said, "I wouldn't move to California—the ocean water is too cold. But I *would* move to Hawaii." My husband agreed without hesitation.

I loved swimming in warm oceans while on vacation, especially with the wildlife, on our numerous trips around the world. Two of the most memorable trips I'd had were to Hawaii, the first with my ex-husband to Kona and the second to Maui with my current husband. Although I loved these visits, it never actually crossed my mind to move to Hawaii.

That night, the talk of moving away from Washington was wishful thinking. My husband and I wanted to become snowbirds when the kids graduated high school, a distant prospect because my son, the youngest of the two, was just finishing fifth grade. My husband, who was affected by seasonal depression, longed to escape the months of gray Washington days in exchange for sunshine. We had visited Mexico, Belize, and Arizona to explore which location would be ideal for our snowbird adventures.

Thoughts of moving to Hawaii kept churning in my mind, despite how illogical the idea was. My husband had finally established himself in his Olympia-based mortgage business, after restarting his life following his divorce. We wondered if he could maintain his referral sources in Washington while building his business in Hawaii. Due to the pandemic, he knew he could work virtually, as he had been successfully doing so for two months.

Career-wise, I had other considerations. My spiritual business was online and geographically independent. My home staging business, which was for sale, could operate remotely with my employees executing the daily tasks. The biggest obstacle to a move was my son, who lived with me the majority of the time after his dad and I divorced. I felt certain his dad wouldn't permit a move across the ocean. Since we weren't planning a move, I didn't focus on the "what ifs."

After a few days, our wishful thinking turned into a general plan to move to Hawaii in a couple of years. As a family, we watched all fourteen seasons of HGTV's *Hawaii Life*, dreaming of a future move. We watched YouTube videos on the history and culture of Hawaii. My excitement about the possibility grew stronger. I started to visualize us living there, feeling how amazing it would be. Signs of Hawaii popped up everywhere around me.

Because my husband did all of his work virtually, a thought crossed our minds: *Why wait a couple of years to move? Why not now?* It seemed impulsive, but every part of my body screamed, "yes," to move to Hawaii as soon as possible. After years of not trusting and following my inner wisdom, I had learned to take the first step when I got a true "yes" from my soul, even when it didn't make sense. We agreed to make the move happen within the year. My head spun with anticipation and excitement.

That summer, we sold off items we wouldn't move with us, as a shipping container would cost as much as purchasing all new furniture. I planned to take only travel artifacts and clothing. The more items that sold, the more real our move became. The momentum built.

Our initial plan was that we would rent a home, so we could get to know the area before choosing where we would purchase. Because we had two cats and a dog, we weren't able to rent (who knew multiple pets would be an issue?). For a moment, I doubted we would be able to move.

With the dire rental market situation, we switched gears and explored purchasing a home. We encountered issues with regards to our employment situation due to me being self-employed and my husband's business being dependent on referrals.

Fortunately, we were able to come up with a plan to make it work. We had to buy the house as a second home, rather than a primary residence like we had originally hoped. We were financially able to purchase a second home in Hawaii. It was now September.

With our funding in place, we narrowed our search to one specific neighborhood, looking at homes online, as Hawaii had a mandatory two-week quarantine for visitors. Our agent shared video tours of two homes, one of which we liked but weren't ready to make an offer. A couple of days later, she called saying that someone submitted an offer on the house we liked, and we would have to act quickly if we had any hopes of getting it. I felt anxious about the prospect of losing that home.

After a brief discussion with my husband, we made the strongest offer we could, knowing the seller had already sent a counteroffer to the first buyer. The seller rescinded the counter in time to accept our offer as is, no counter-offer necessary. The house was ours! Excitement and relief coursed through my body. We were moving to Hawaii by the end of the year!

The loan process flowed with grace and ease, and our house closed before Thanksgiving. Then we listed our home in Washington. I had pre-emptively prepared the home for the market, so we were ready the day after closing on our Hawaiian home. In two days, we had fifteen offers, with most over the asking price. We accepted the strongest offer, and set the closing date for December 28, with us flying the family to Hawaii on December 30.

The biggest challenge became my son's living situation. Throughout the process of purchasing a home, we held on to the hopes that his father would let him move to Hawaii with us. My daughter, who has a different father than my son, would be able to move with no issues.

In our early dreaming stages, my son's dad seemed more open to the idea, as it would be a great experience for him. I had doubts that would continue when the move became real, and I was correct. As soon as we closed on our Hawaii home, my son's dad turned 180 degrees and said that he would not be going to Hawaii.

I was crushed, but not surprised. My son was angry at his father for saying no and angry at me for moving away from him. He blamed me for divorcing his father six years earlier, still not fully grasping why it was for the best for all of us.

I wasn't in a financial or energetic position to fight in court, so I acquiesced. In talking with a couple of my psychic friends, they reassured me that it would likely not be a permanent situation. That gave me some hope.

My son stayed with us for the first two weeks in Hawaii before returning to Washington for school. It was a challenging time, as he was still angry and lashed out at me daily. It took a couple of months for him to talk to me on the phone after his return.

He came to visit for Spring Break, and it was a completely different experience. We had plenty of bonding time, exploring the island and ocean together. I shared my love of snorkeling and introduced him to my favorite animals, the manta rays. On our first snorkel experience, he reached over hugged me and gave me a heart symbol with his hands. I melted.

We have lived in our Hawaii home now for four months. I wake up with a smile on my face, reminding myself that this is real, not a dream. We are well on our way to establishing ourselves here in business and friendships. My son remains in Washington State with his dad, but I trust he will be here with us one day. We talk on the phone a few times a week and have scheduled his summer visit. Although my mama's heart is sad, I know without a doubt I made the correct decision for me and my family, living our Hawaiian life.

Reflection

What does the word "home" mean to you?

_____

_____

_____

_____

Is there a place you feel called to live, but aren't? What about that place feels like home to you?

_____

_____

_____

_____

Who in your life feels like home to you and how does that knowing impact your experience?

_____

_____

_____

_____

17

Finding Maya and Myself

SARAH BREEN

*O*nly one hour into our ten-hour car ride to Pennsylvania and I was riddled with stress. We had managed to pull together enough money to get us there and back for a friend's wedding. It was just the two of us, and missing our one-year-old son, we talked at length. I still don't know how I ended up with my husband; his calm voice penetrated the silence as I was sinking further into the passenger seat. I always felt as if everything was my fault. My jobs were unreliable, as I moved from small business to small business in hopes that something would pan out over time. Depression was a regular knock on my door. We spoke about what needed to change and how we could do it together. As the hours went by, we bounced between our normal sarcastic playfulness and the serious changes we needed to make. We have always been a strong couple with "get off my brainwave" comments being frequent. He knew I was teetering on another breakdown. I met my husband shortly after I attempted suicide, he knows me from my lowest points in life.

"Ugh, you used to drive like this for college how often?" I said, stretching uncomfortably. He grinned at my avoidance.

We arrived at the hotel around 2 p.m., somewhere deep in the mountains where churches were conveniently located next to the smoke shops and convenience stores. Desperately needing to stretch, a gust of frigid air shocked me. Tired, cold, and hungry we made our way through the hotel to our room. Stressed about finances, career choices, and our future I needed to meditate and attempt to pull myself together. I splashed cold water on my face, kicking off my shoes, and plopping on the bed with ear buds. I randomly chose a track on YouTube. Drums and rattles filled my ears, and I was paralyzed where I sat. Falling into the Earth feeling my way around the cave, smelling the rich fertile soil of the Mother. Coming upon a flickering flame in the distance I sensed a deep pull from my heart forward. It began to get bigger and bigger until heat from the fire blazed on my face. A being was on the other side.

"Find Maya," it shouted. With a jolt I found myself back on the hotel bed, dazed and confused. I looked down to see what I had got myself into and found I stumbled onto a *journey* track. "What is a journey and who is Maya?" I frantically searched for my laptop in hopes of finding answers. Articles of journeying, shamanism, and then I found Maya—an actual person who was only three hours away from my residence. I quickly emailed her explaining what had happened. She responded within twenty minutes suggesting we meet. I closed my laptop and exhaled with relief.

Stepping into a small spiritual shop where incenses and sage fill the air, I was beckoned to sit at the circle with an altar of crystals, power objects, and furs in the center. Maya asked each person for two words that described themselves. I was frantically trying to think of words when "curious and stubborn" blurted out of my mouth. While thinking those words together sounded like I failed the test, she smiled warmly. She had the best smile, sitting in her comfortable clothes, random tattoos, teal streaks through her dark brown hair, and always plenty of snacks at her side. For years I drove monthly to visit her. Our circles shrunk over time the deeper we went; growing close through frequent phone conversations, in person meetings, and emails as I worked through the invisible territory.

Maya taught me how to be one with myself, honor my process, and be in a partnership with Spirit. I knew my emotional mind was more than I could handle on my own, so I had to trust in my process, to not abandon or avoid myself anymore. As the years progressed, I mastered journeying, elemental kinship, astral traveling, past life regressions, dream walking, ancestors, and ultimately losing myself in time and space to come back home more alive than before.

She encouraged my curiosity as the ancestors called my name. With my drum in hand, I took my journey up to the realm of our beloved ancestors, with deep respect stepping up to grandfather fire calling out to those of my bloodline to come forward. Hand after hand reached through the fire. They broke out in cheers by my side, I heard "she's still alive" and "she came home." Uncertain if the "she's still alive" comment was because I've been a project for them or was this a normal thing to happen? The cheers stopped as another hand reached through the fire. They nudged me to take it. A man about six foot two with a cut chin, strong shoulders, and a stern look came through the fire. My uncomfortable humor broke the silence as I invited them to come back home to my altar. They each agreed happily till we got to this man. "You know you really don't have to come down, you can stay here it's really nice and cozy up here." He nodded without a word walking past me to join the others. "Oh boy... wait till Maya hears about this character."

Aflred (pronounced a-fled) has become a force to be reckoned with. One who will stop me dead in my tracks and protect my heart at all costs. "Your sarcasm needs an adjustment. Honor your heart and pay attention!" is his daily reminder. Even with entanglements with those I held karma with from previous lives he would step in with force. Similar to the seatbelt arm a parent would give you in the passenger seat, he would forcefully pull me back from engaging further. The wind would get knocked out of me when I chose not to listen to my heart. Maya always reminded me to listen not with your ears but with the flow of your spirit. She would smirk as I regurgitated my experiences with "That is yet another initiation you just walked through. Welcome dear one!" I learned to not ask too many questions with big statements like that.

On a chilly October day, the autumn sun peeked through the oak trees as my two boys ran joyously in the backyard. I sat with my back against the trees as they sang and swayed in the wind. Yellow, purple, and orange leaves danced to the Earth, embracing the season of shedding. Taking a deep breath, I felt a shift in consciousness; something was missing but it felt expansive. A text message alerted me to Maya's passing unexpectedly from an eight-month battle with cancer. I felt my world crashing around me. Our journey had only begun, and I had so much to learn. But just as a mama bird pushes her baby out of the nest, I had to have the courage to spread my wings and fly.

I knew in my heart that death is not the end; it is another beginning. That night I opened sacred space with grandfather fire to honor Maya for showing me something I couldn't see in myself. Then I finally said "YES" to Spirit. I said YES from my entire being. Feeling everything at once, dropping to my knees as all of my beloved ancestors, lineages, and Maya witnessed what was unfolding. A voice from within cried out, "YES, Spirit! I am here for my destiny. To break the chains of the unresolved patterns of the past freeing our ancestors. I am a beacon of light for our future. A beacon that moves through the darkness to bring light to the forgotten. I say YES tonight being witnessed by all that stand here, visible and invisible, to free the way for our greatest becoming." My inhale affirmed my flight as the cold air rushed into my body for the first time. "Yes, I am here, Yes I am strong, Yes I am worthy, and Yes I am one."

I think back on my journey and wouldn't change a single moment. Our journey will align us with our greatest lessons to find beauty. I know who I am and remain curious when shining light in our darkness. Shedding what no longer serves us to fully embody our authentic selves. Holding courage in the face of fears. Committing to my souls' journey by saying yes without knowing what it is. Embracing my medicine that calls from my soul to bring to the world. I never was abandoned; I was only afraid of embodying my light and shining it as I was designed to do. I honor all who have come before us while maintaining a sacred relationship with Spirit so our children can be today what their authentic selves came here to create.

Reflection

In what ways has fear stopped you from shining your light?

_____

_____

_____

_____

What recurring situations and emotions have you not yet acknowledged and how are they holding you back?

_____

_____

_____

_____

How has meditation opened your curiosity, shaped your destiny, and challenged your spirituality?

_____

_____

_____

_____

CHAPTER TWO

SELF
Reimagined

The Healing Power of Self-Compassion

KELLEY GRIMES, MSW

*L*ooking over the beautiful catalog that arrived in the mail, I longed to attend a workshop at Esalen. Since I was a teenager, I dreamt of visiting the retreat center I first noticed as I drove along the Big Sur coastline. Perched overlooking the crashing waves of the Pacific Ocean and nestled in the forest, Esalen beckoned me, yet going there seemed out of reach. In addition to its stunning location, it had developed a mystique created by so many of my most beloved authors, philosophers, psychologists, and artists who had been teaching there for the last sixty years. Its inspiring mission was to work toward the realization of a more just, creative, and sustainable world. I felt deeply called to be there.

The advent of my becoming an empty nester coincided with my fiftieth birthday, and it seemed a perfect time to finally give myself the gift of a self-nurturing retreat at Esalen. After spending a lifetime nurturing and caring for others, I found my sense of identity and purpose had become inextricably entwined with my caregiving role. As my youngest daughter Zoey prepared to leave for college, I wondered what this next stage of my life would look like. I struggled to make sense of the myriad of emotions I felt and the excitement of new possibilities opening in my life. This led me to ponder the existential questions of who I wanted to be, and what I wanted to do with my time now that my daily parenting responsibilities were ending.

Going on a retreat felt like a compassionate way to explore these profound questions and create space to reimagine my life. To my delight, Esalen offered a workshop called "Leading with Relational Mindfulness: Regenerating Ourselves and the World" the week of my birthday. This workshop seemed made for me and I was overjoyed! I registered in advance to reserve my place and invited some dear friends to join me. I felt so proud of myself for prioritizing time for me and empowering my husband to help our daughter pack for college. The retreat was scheduled to end on my birthday, and we planned that my husband and daughter would pick me up on the way to Santa Cruz so we could celebrate together, and then help Zoey get settled into her dorm room.

All the plans were coming together beautifully until torrential rains caused major flooding, landslides, and bridge closures, and Esalen had to close for six months. Blessedly and miraculously, they were able to reopen a few weeks before my retreat was scheduled. The drive through the mountains to get to the retreat center was harrowing as Highway 1 remained closed in places, but the moment we arrived at Esalen it felt like I had come home.

The physical beauty surrounding me was breathtaking, with amazing views of the ocean, forests of magnificent trees, thriving gardens, creeks falling into a waterfall at the circular meditation room, and the lush mountains looming behind the retreat center. I immediately felt deeply nurtured and rejuvenated in this magical place, and as a result I began to realize that making a commitment to live my dream was nourishing my own value and worth.

The experience felt even more nurturing as the vision that had drawn me to Esalen for years was now embodied in the workshop I attended. Nina Simons and Deborah Eden Tull, the workshop's facilitators, said, "*In this time of so much change, we are all called to be leaders.*" They invited us to practice a kinder, more compassionate, and inclusive form of leadership where we lead from our *whole* selves, honoring our need to nurture ourselves, while advancing the life-enhancing changes the world called for. They encouraged us to show up with purpose, love, and whole-heartedness in every area of our lives, and took us through many exercises throughout the workshop, to deepen our ability to do so.

This remarkable Esalen experience had self-nurturing woven into every aspect. Each day I hiked, meditated in the circular meditation room under the waterfall, practiced yoga, soaked in the mineral waters under the stars, ate nourishing organic food, enjoyed time with friends, and journaled. I felt deeply rejuvenated by the beauty all around me. I unplugged from email and social media and found taking a technology fast felt both liberating and restorative. Being present in this new way allowed me to deeply connect with myself and the other workshop participants, rather than be distracted by responsibilities of home and work. This precious time allowed me to culti-vate a new loving and compassionate relationship with myself that was pro-foundly healing and has rippled out into every area of my life.

I learned invaluable lessons from the wise and empowering facilitators and other beautiful participants, about the healing power of transparency and deep listening, the profound courage required to be vulnerable, and to show up authentically, how cultivating self-awareness in community amplifies the impact, and the gift of pausing to reconnect with ourselves, our breath, and our bodies throughout the day. I came to understand that spending this time with myself allowed my self-compassion to blossom and deepened my ability to respond to my life experiences with kindness, tenderness, and as a loving friend. Most powerfully, I learned how to compassionately come home to myself again and again, empowering me to reimagine my life and express more of who I am in the world without fear of failure.

Learning to treat myself like a dear friend has transformed my life from the inside out. My high expectations of myself and critical thinking have decreased over time as curiosity and non-judgment inspire more of how I perceive myself. Now I give myself so much more grace around mistakes and see each mistake as an opportunity to learn and grow, reinforcing my growth mindset. Self-compassion has nurtured my belief that life is about progress not perfection and has liberated me in so many ways. In this healing process, I have been able to recognize deep hurts that I was holding onto and transform them with tenderness, curiosity, and forgiveness. I am now able to love and appreciate myself deeply and feel profound gratitude for everything in my life. And miraculously, the self-directed energy of love, kindness, and compassion has allowed me to share more of that energy in the world, which feels deeply purposeful and meaningful. After giving myself permission to live this dream and cultivate more self-compassion, I had the courage to write the book I have dreamed about writing for ten years: *The Art of Self-Nurturing: A Field Guide to Living with More Peace, Joy, and Meaning.*

Spending five life changing days at Esalen provided me a cellular mem-ory of feeling deeply nourished, cherished, and nurtured by myself! Even as I processed the profound sadness of missing my daughter Zoey after I returned home, I felt a deep sense of calm and peace as I tended to myself with love and compassion through the process. And even though I have been on a self-nurturing journey for years, the Esalen experience deepened my relationship with myself and inspired me to reimagine my life each day by expressing more creativity, love, empathy, joy, and gratitude in the world. Understanding the healing power of self-compassion has been revolutionary and has been the ultimate antidote to living in this stressful and challenging world. Choosing self-compassion empowers me every day to embody and radiate who I want to be in the world and from that my gratitude flows.

As Deborah Eden Toll reminded us throughout the workshop, "*Awareness is the subtlest form of love. Be sure you give yourself the gift of your own kind awareness.*"

Reflection

Is there a dream you are yearning to manifest?

_____

_____

_____

_____

What would it look like to treat yourself like your own best friend?

_____

_____

_____

_____

What difference could self-compassion make in your life

_____

_____

_____

_____

Mirror Reflections

ROBIN EATON

*G*lancing in the mirror, I started to cry; I couldn't bear to see the anguish in my own eyes. Sobbing in desperation, I slumped to the bathroom floor. I didn't know what to do. I didn't want to live in this agony, and I couldn't seem to change it. I looked at the bottle of pills and considered checking out. I felt trapped in a nightmare. I wanted to wake up as someone else.

Violet pressed her cold nose into my cheek. Ronin whined and licked my tears. I hugged my dogs close and then pulled myself together for work. I was a Federal Officer who specialized in child pornography investigations. Making a difference was my reason to live. I could help others, even if I couldn't help myself. Work was my bizarre refuge.

I sat in my office reviewing videos, spanning a decade, of over twenty victims—all abused by the same man. Drugged women being used like rag dolls, toddlers who grew to be school children—all captured on film as they desperately attempted evasion from their inevitable abuse. The vacant looks in the children's eyes haunted me. Vomit rose in my throat, and I ran to the bathroom to purge.

That case was my breaking point, the final straw in my already fractured world. I crumpled into myself, afraid to sleep because of the night terrors. I vanished from social events because of the panic attacks. I couldn't be intimate without video images looping in my head. I saw potential threats everywhere. When I looked in the mirror, I saw despair looking back. I hated that most of all.

With trepidation, I sought help. My shrink was impressed with how I held myself together considering the level of vicarious trauma I was exposed to on a daily basis. She wasn't sure what she could offer me. I raged inside, trapped in a dark well by secrets I couldn't allow out. If I did, she'd have to report me. They'd take away my gun, my job, my lifeline. Ironic, my career was both torturer and savior. She gave me a diagnosis: PTSD, and a prescription of no more child porn cases. I walked away defeated and alone.

My prescription got me transferred to a supervision unit. I felt punished for speaking up. I believed management was setting me up to be fired and I fought to hold onto the one place I felt worthy. The anger was exactly what I needed. Battling to prove myself in a new arena felt invigorating—a new distraction—a band-aid on the stab wound to my soul. The relief was temporary.

When the dream came, it felt so real. Terror flooded my body, dumping adrenaline, but I had nowhere to run. I was trapped in a cage, listening to his footsteps coming for me. He was going to skin me alive like the last one. The smell of her burnt flesh hung in the air. Like an animal caught in a snare, I gnawed my wrist. Better to bleed out than suffer the same fate as my torturer's previous victim.

I woke disoriented, feeling the cold weight in my hand as I raised the gun to my head. Realization sank in as my bedroom materialized. I had almost shot myself. When had the lines become so blurred? When did I lose my mind? I couldn't trust myself.

I found a new shrink. She seemed more traumatized by my story than I was. I witnessed horror grow in her eyes as I spoke, and I felt her withdraw. I stopped talking and she quit asking questions. I left, dejected. It had taken every ounce of courage and humility I had to reach out for help again, only to have my hope crushed; annihilated.

I was a fraud. Every day, I advised my clients to live full lives. Meanwhile, my standing Friday night date was with paperwork at the office. My friendships faded away as my paranoia and depression grew. I let my hobbies go. If I wasn't at work, I was isolated at home. I hated my life and who I'd become.

I immersed myself in self-help and found a little spark of hope. I scrambled to keep it alive. I traveled to Denver for a conference, needing to be in a room with my new mentors and people who thought like them. If that couldn't help me, nothing would.

I listened to Anita Moorjani describe her return from death and it struck me like a sucker punch. I wasn't afraid of dying; I flirted with death on a daily basis. I was afraid to live. In that moment, I recognized that nearly every choice I made was rooted in fear. Fear of being hurt, of disappointment, of failure. I was afraid to live life as me.

What if I made choices from love? What would that look like? Did I have the courage? What if I tried it for just one day? What if I stopped hiding and listened to my intuition? I tucked suicide in my back pocket in case it didn't work out.

I took a deep breath. My heart felt lighter. It was like being handed a map with a faint route traced from despair to happiness. This time I cried tears of hope. I left the conference in a fragile bubble of bliss. Praying it wouldn't pop and plunge me to new depths.

I spent the following week alone in the Rocky Mountains. I stretched my limits hiking Ypsilon Mountain. I nurtured myself in a spa tub under the stars. I listened to my heart and let myself dream. I looked inside for answers and my intuition heeded the call.

My niece was born that week. I hated missing that moment with my sister, but I knew what I needed. I wanted to be someone my niece could look up to which meant I had to get right with myself. I stopped thinking of myself as a victim and I looked in the mirror with clear eyes. I recovered my soul and my connection to Source. I went through a birth of my own, like the phoenix rising from the ashes, wondering if I really could fly.

It was a beginning. I returned home with a delicate thread of connection to the heart of life and a desire to experience it fully. I strengthened the link by listening to my intuition. I stopped allowing myself to be bullied at work. If I wasn't afraid of death, why should I fear getting fired? I set uncompromising boundaries; I reclaimed my time. Then I had to figure out what to do with that time. I felt like a toddler awkwardly exploring the world.

I attended a psychic fair for an aura photo. I loved the marriage between tech and the unseen world. As I waited my turn, I found myself asking all sorts of questions about the equipment and how they learned to read the photos. Before I knew it, I was spending crazy money buying the latest aura technology.

I felt like a little kid with a new puppy when the camera arrived. I fumbled through the set up and reached for the instruction book explaining what the aura colors meant. My intuition told me to throw it away. I rebelled. Books are sacred. I couldn't throw it out. How would I use this fancy equipment without the instructions? My intuition stayed steady. *Throw the book away. Trust yourself. You already know this. You've been reading energy your whole life.* For the next two weeks, I invested time playing with the camera. Somewhere therein, I found my prayers answered. I was happy.

Nerves jangling, I booked a booth at a fair. It was time to come out of the psychic closet. I felt like I just branded my forehead, and everyone would call me crazy. But my intuition was driving the show and taking me along for the ride.

The first person approached for a reading. Currents of electricity ran up my arms and legs. Once we started, my whole being quieted, and my awareness narrowed. I was locked in a bubble with my client, reading the energy and lines of destiny. Knowing poured through me as I trusted myself, and Spirit. The day flew by. I looked in the mirror that night and saw a smile in my eyes. My soul purred with satisfaction.

Within months, I left law enforcement to start my adventure as a spiritual entrepreneur. I was being sought out and paid for being me—exactly who I used to fear and hide from. I was sharing hope, something I thought I'd never find. For the first time in a long time, I felt at home in my own skin. I liked the path I was on and who I'd become.

Reflection

How has witnessing trauma impacted your life and how did you move through it?

_____

_____

_____

_____

In what ways have previous experiences brought you home to yourself?

_____

_____

_____

_____

Are there places in your life where you can release past trauma?

_____

_____

_____

_____

What's Wrong with Me?

CATHY CASTEEL

"Just be patient. The right person is out there for you. Don't settle for less. It is worth the wait."

If I heard those words once more, I would explode. Under my breath, I mutter, "It is easy for you to say because you are already married, you found someone who wanted to spend the rest of his life with you, you just don't get it." While the other voice said, *What is wrong with you, no one wants to spend their life with you?*

When I was thirteen years old, I had my first boyfriend, Richard. Even though, technically, I wasn't allowed boyfriends at the time, my mom made an exception since Richard was known to our family. I felt special and pretty because Richard had chosen me.

Then I discovered he was seeing other girls. *What's wrong with me?* became the question I played on a loop in my mind. I naturally assumed his lack of interest was due to some fault of mine because I wasn't fulfilling his needs or something. Looking back, I see now that I inherited this thinking pattern from my mom and her response to how my dad treated her.

For twenty years, I repeated toxic relationships because that was all I knew. My heart got broken many times and the ugly question kept coming back, *What is wrong with me that no one wants to spend their life with me?*

When I met a man who treated me like a queen, his gentlemanly ways were foreign to me and I thought, *This guy is too nice to me. There must be something wrong with him.* I purposely remained distant and refused to invest myself fully in the relationship because he was different from the others and I didn't know what to do.

Eventually I met Jonathan whom I dated for more than seven years. I thought he was "the one." From the beginning of our relationship, I did whatever it took to make it work because I believed that was what you did for someone you loved. I was tired of ending up broken hearted, so I gave everything to the relationship. I lost every single piece of myself during the course of those seven years. I hid junk food so I wouldn't get lectured about why I should not be eating it. I starved myself to lose weight just to make him happy. I walked on eggshells while my unhappiness grew; and even then, walking away didn't feel like an option.

One day, Jonathan asked me to marry him. *It had finally happened!* There mustn't be anything wrong with me because he wanted to spend the rest of his life with me. My unhappiness temporarily evaporated as I threw myself into planning our wedding, while he didn't provide any input or feedback on his side. The day I told him I was going to look at dresses with my mom was the day my happiness evaporated.

Jonathan said, "I really don't want to get married. I just bought you the ring to cheer you up."

Are you for real? I mean, you buy a girl flowers or take her to dinner to cheer her up. You don't ask someone to marry you TO CHEER HER UP! I felt empty; hollowed out. Fortunately, I had to go away for four months for a class, which was a perfect time to get some distance. This distance was a blessing because I realized how much I had morphed myself for someone who didn't really want to marry me.

I left the relationship with the same question I'd been asking myself at thirteen, *What is wrong with me?* Over the next eight years, I dated, thinking I had learned my lessons, but those relationships were short and unfulfilling. I didn't realize that the question I kept asking myself led me down that destructive path.

One day, I sat in my house feeling alone and tired, desperately wanting my life to change, when I heard a voice say, "How long are you going to keep doing this to yourself? How can you expect someone to love you if you don't love yourself?" Hearing those words was like an awakening from a long sleep to the realization that I must change. I had a hunger to find out who I really was, and what I truly wanted.

I chose not to date for the next four years, embarking on a path of self-discovery and self-love instead. I dove deep into my faith and said to the Divine, "I know you put me on this earth to do your work, and I am done fighting what it is you put me here to do." I explored what I truly wanted in life and focused on doing things that brought me joy. I served others while still spending time on myself.

During this time of self-discovery, I learned how to love myself. I practiced being comfortable with myself by going to movies alone, eating out by myself, reading books on self-development and self-reflection. Also, I realized that the amazing contributions I brought to a relationship like kindness, humor, gentleness, and joy, would *complement* a life partner rather than trying to complete him. I made the choice not to settle for anything less than what my heart really wanted. I made a commitment to being my authentic self; to no longer giving my soul, worth, or dreams away to someone else in exchange for love.

Those years felt like eternity as I worked to discover who the real me was, loving that beautiful little girl inside of me who I had ignored for so long. The war that had raged inside finally quieted and, for the first time, I experienced internal peace. I made a list of non-negotiables that I wanted in my soulmate and waited for the person the Divine had chosen for me. I thought, *This is a tough list, am I really worthy of such a special person?* But whenever negative thoughts or self-doubt arose, I chose to put my faith in the Divine who would tell me, "Trust me and you will see." And I did.

In October 2008, I went on my first date in four years. That night, I met Robert, my forever date, my soulmate, and my best friend in the world, at a restaurant we both agreed upon. Prior to that date we spent every night for three weeks, talking on the phone for hours and getting to know each other deeply.

We would laugh a lot while also making time for the serious conversations about what we both wanted out of our lives. The relationship flowed with such ease and there was a really deep connection from the beginning. It was foreign to me and I doubted myself. The doubt sparked me to have a conversation with one of my sisters.

She said, "Cathy, he is different and maybe that is the point. You need to date someone different from who you have dated in the past."

I was deeply grateful for that conversation because it alleviated those
unworthy feelings that kept showing up despite all the work I'd done on myself. I decided to trust and see where it took me. I pulled out my list of non-negotiables—noticing that he met all of them; even the ones I thought would be asking too much. Apparently, the Divine knew my true worth more than I was willing to believe.

Now, as we approach our fourteenth anniversary, I feel so blessed and grateful for the journey I undertook. Because if I had not learned, I would not have been able to recognize the gift that was placed in front of me. Now I feel comfortable being treated like a queen. I have learned how to love deeply and unconditionally, and how to be authentic with myself and my partner.

Before my mom died, I thanked her for what she had taught me about giving myself grace and I understood that we make the best decisions we can based on the information we have at the time. If I had not hit rock bottom and invested in myself, I wouldn't have been in a place to receive the incredible gift the Divine had for me: My husband.

Learning to trust myself, learning to love myself, and learning that I was responsible for my worth, has transformed my life. And I forward that gift by helping other women to do the same. The Divine has remained with me the whole way along this beautiful journey of transformation.

Reflection

In what ways has believing you weren't worthy impacted your life?

_____

_____

_____

_____

What places in your life can you invite more grace in and how would that impact you?

_____

_____

_____

_____

What patterns have you inherited from your family and do they serve you?

_____

_____

_____

_____

Life Outside of the Box

KRIS GROTH

A wheezing sound emerged from my throat. My chest and throat constricted. Driving home from my weekend job after completing my last day before being furloughed, the difficulty breathing came out of nowhere, or so it seemed. Asthma? I've always had allergies, but never asthma. Maybe it was a result of the pneumonia I'd had. I coughed, in an attempt to open things up, but the constriction persisted. Then as quickly as it started, it eased up, and I could breathe again. Even though it felt like a long time, the wheezing only lasted a minute or two before my breathing returned to normal.

The side job was essential when my in-person business was shut down by the governor six weeks into the pandemic. We used the funds to cover expenses. What was I going to do?

Hopelessness at the impossibility of the situation overwhelmed me. The money just wasn't there. Once again, the asthma returned, making it hard for me to take a breath. I tried meditating and going for walks, but nothing seemed to help. Fear of the future loomed heavily around me.

Old beliefs and buried fears around money and poverty hovered front and center in my mind. A lack mindset had driven my life for so many years without my awareness. The pandemic unearthed those hidden fears and brought them to light. No more ignoring or pretending, the time had arrived to look at the shadows and face the dark and ugly within me.

When I was one year old, a tornado destroyed our home and all of our possessions. While I don't remember this happening, the trauma planted seeds of lack and poverty in my subconscious that have continued to grow ever since. The insidious beliefs that "others can have all that but not me," "I don't deserve more," "it never works out for me," "no matter how hard I try, it is never enough," and "hold onto what you have because it can be gone in an instant," controlled my actions and decisions from behind the scenes. I thought this was just my lot in life, the way it has always been and would always be for me.

These old beliefs tried to protect me from hurt and disappointment, but actually they kept me tucked away in a tiny little box, one that had become stifling and uncomfortable. Within this box, I became who others expected me to be. I kept the peace and didn't make waves, and I didn't try for anything more. From the outside, the box looked fine, but inside it was confining and suffocating. It just didn't fit, I couldn't breathe.

For years I worked to heal past wounds, learned to love and accept myself, and cleared away old baggage. I set intentions for the life I wanted and prayed daily for miracles to come my way. Still, I felt hopelessly stuck. Would anything ever change for the better?

My go-to sacred space at home is outside in the gazebo, lying in my hammock. I snuggled into the hammock's cradle and called in my angels, envisioning myself being surrounded by light. I felt their presence, and a sense of peace enveloped me. I asked for help, guidance, and clarity.

Within my blissful relaxed state, a knowing came over me that everything would be okay. The angels guided me to focus on self-care, whatever would feed my soul and make me feel happy. Surrender and trust it.

Self-care and spiritual connection became my new full-time job. I developed a daily routine that included expressing gratitude, journaling, meditation, and walks in nature. I dug out my watercolors and started painting again. Inspiration flowed for my next book. Through it all, my angels remained at my side.

A shocking realization struck me that with the shutdown, the universe actually brought me exactly what I asked for. I wanted to have my weekends free—and my weekend job was furloughed. Something needed to shift in my work, but I didn't know how or what. I felt nudged to expand my online business and do more teaching, coaching, and writing. The desire to have more time for creative projects and doing things that I loved could also be satisfied. It brought what I didn't know I needed...deep healing and change.

The pandemic shined a light on what needed to heal, and I recognized I had a chance to heal issues around money and self-worth that had plagued me my entire life. For the first time, I had unlimited time to work on myself without the distraction of a job. What a perfect opportunity to utilize the various healing tools and techniques I had gathered throughout the years.

After intensely working on shifting my mindset and healing my relationship to money, as well as surrendering to the divine and trusting that everything would work out, miracles began occurring. Money flowed in from unexpected places. Opportunities popped up left and right for both my husband and me. The angels and the universe showed me that everything really was working out for me. I could breathe again.

A lightbulb went off, and it became crystal clear that my issues with money were never about the numbers but reflected what I felt I deserved. Shifting my beliefs of self-worth allowed me to step into the divine flow...of abundance, inspiration and joy.

My focus each day centered on connecting with my angels, raising my vibration, and doing what made me happy. With no goal in mind, I took advantage of this unexpected blessing to do whatever I wanted and to allow myself to just be. As a result, I experienced a freedom I never before thought possible.

One morning, I woke up feeling fully vibrant and excited for no reason at all. There was nothing special planned; it was just an ordinary day. Joy permeated my entire being. All day long, I laughed like a giddy schoolgirl. Energy radiated through my body making me feel tingly all over. No matter what I did—computer work, meditation, cooking dinner—the buzzing joyous feeling continued. Even cleaning a disastrous kitchen cupboard didn't kill this natural high.

The next day, my energy was still positive and upbeat, though less intense. It occurred to me that the high I'd been feeling was a result of raising my vibration. I was living in the energy of joy. I knew then that I didn't want to go back to the way things had been before.

Deep reflection and journaling helped me clarify what was happening. My new vibration aligned with light, joy, and ease. That's what I wanted more of. Whatever was out of alignment felt heavy, draining, and stressful. I was ready to release those feelings. I envisioned a life that lit me up inside, one in alignment with my light and truth. Anything that didn't resonate with that vibration felt wrong.

How amazing to be in a place where I had the time, space, and opportunity to not only dream about how I wanted my life to be, but with everything shut down, I could implement those changes now. Gone was the fear and despair of all that was changing. Turns out, embracing the fears was an answer to so many prayers.

What surprised me most was how, throughout this time of unprecedented upheaval and uncertainty, I felt calm, contented, and more at peace than ever. I finally envisioned an abundant future and knew, deep within, it was coming for me.

My angels guided me not only to create a new way of doing business, but a whole new way of being and showing up in the world. Parts of me were revealed that had been hidden far too long, and I felt like a whole new person.

I can't tell you how good it feels to get to know myself, and to see what I am capable of. It isn't always easy. I still bump up against old programming and beliefs that try to put me back in a box and contain me, but now that I have emerged and felt the sun on my face and wind under my wings, there is no going back. Whatever comes next, I know I am meant to fly! I am free to be me, and it feels amazing!

Reflection

What old beliefs run in the back of your mind and keep you small?

_____

_____

_____

_____

What can you do each day to raise your vibration and bring in more joy?

_____

_____

_____

_____

What changes can you make in your life to be more in alignment with your truth? What would you let go of? What do you want more of?

_____

_____

_____

_____

Reclaiming My Red Thread

CRYSTAL COCKERHAM

I sat, just off the beach, on one of the lawn swings outside the retreat center, on a partly sunny June afternoon. A cool breeze came off Lake Huron, its water lapping upon the shore steadily, echoing the storm of my thoughts and emotions.

I had come to the retreat with more than twenty other women, for the first of two, weekend-long, retreats that were part of a nine-month program of Sacred Women's work. I knew no one there. Despite being in uncharted territory, I had no questions about my call to be part of it, or the knowing in my soul that I was exactly where I needed to be.

Earlier that day, we had broken up our circle into groups of four to recount our first moon flow stories, stemming from a pre-retreat homework assignment. Journaling about my first period brought up lots of feelings, mostly of disappointment at not remembering much. The only thing I could remember is that I was nine years old and in the fourth grade. When it came time for me to share, I told them what I remembered: my mom calling to me from the bathtub to tell me that our neighbor had gotten a library book for me to read and it was on her dresser. She told me to read it and to let her know if I had any questions.

The second part of our pre-retreat assignment was to imagine and record how we would have wanted our first moon flow to have been celebrated. Listening to the others' stories triggered my old feelings of being singled out and denied acceptance. I was no longer stuck in my head trying to remember.

My first moon flow wasn't celebrated by my family. There was no acknowledgement of being ushered into the next phase of maturity. It seemed as though I was supposed to act like nothing was happening. There were three or four years where I didn't feel like I belonged anywhere. I felt the loss of my childhood.

If that wasn't bad enough, when I was eleven years old, problems with my cycle began. What sixth grader has a full-on, heavy flow, painful period every other week? I hadn't been ready to start my period when I was nine, so I definitely wasn't prepared for the countless doctor's appointments that lay before me. I had no older siblings and none of my friends could share their experiences because they hadn't had them yet. Even so, I knew something was wrong. I didn't understand what was happening or why. And I was scared.

Hearing the other women's stories, all the shame, anger and fear I hadn't processed in my youth rose to the surface like a tsunami, sweeping me away with its power. Memories of my mother sharing openly about my challenges—and loudly—in doctors' waiting rooms, at large family gatherings, with her friends, in front of my friends—and the utter embarrassment flooded through me once again. All the appointments, my mother's lack of consideration, and my own physical discomfort left me feeling as though I were broken, not good enough, and unloved.

I felt robbed of one of the most beautiful aspects of womanhood: acknowledgement, and celebration of a holy, sacred rite! I had nothing to be ashamed of and everything to celebrate.

All my circle experience had led me to that moment. I had a choice: stay upset, be a victim forever, and continuing to carry the shame, or, to take my power back. I felt both devastated and upset.

As I sat on the lawn swing at the retreat center, the dam broke, and I sobbed.

My mentor, Carolyn, helped me understand that the medical problems with my moon flow were my body's way of rejecting the shame I felt over being a woman. At last: the mother wound I had gone there to heal was undeniable. The cycle would end with me.

After all, being a mother was in fact a miracle for me, an absolute blessing. There was no way that there was room within my body, mind, heck, in my consciousness to carry that duality of both shame and unconditional love any longer.

I took my power back, starting with honoring and loving my body. As I moved through the sacred space held for me that weekend, I physically experienced and mentally processed a rebirth. My abdomen swelled and I had menstrual cramping—all of which was shocking and surreal because I'd had a complete hysterectomy ten years earlier. My body processed and released generational wounds as though I were that young girl again.

The intense a-ha's that came to me as I reflected back (through a lens of wisdom and new-to-me teachings) on that tender time of my youth, reconciled and healed my wounds. I grabbed hold of and reclaimed my power, declaring all the shame, embarrassment, and hiding was over, done, banished, and no longer welcome. Normally, this kind of work happens over a period of months or years. For me, it happened in the space of one weekend. Then came the work of integrating and embodying my newly found and claimed truth.

It wasn't easy to embrace and love those missing parts of me and my story. I had to fully embody all the teachings, and trainings I had received until then, as an energy healer and coach, as well as plunge into the unknown.

Some people learn a foreign language gradually while others choose an immersive experience. By consciously choosing to take my power back, embrace the Divine Feminine within me and own it like a Goddess, I had unknowingly chosen the immersive experience. My ascension shifted from turbo to warp speed. The tapestry of my life to date was re-woven; transformed.

That Red Thread found a new place, prominent, poised, and powerful. That younger me who experienced shame and embarrassment finally had her voice heard and I was reunited with her. After all, I had the miraculous gift of physical motherhood and unconditional love for my children. I knew how to give love to others; it was time to give it to and receive it from myself.

My soul's purpose was alive and pulsing inside me with its own heartbeat. I learned to trust myself and follow my intuitive senses or continue to face harsh and painful lessons until I did so; floundering like a baby learning to walk. Getting bruised over and over, and over again. I needed to pay attention to my emotions, my truth, and to live my life. It was not my place to take on the burdens and wounds of others.

My place was either to claim my inner healer and visionary aspects or continue living an empty life.

I reconciled with the younger me, who had fought so hard, for so long; through tremendous physical pain—trying everything she could to retain her reproductive organs. I would not be here today if she hadn't. I am stronger and more seated in my power, my sacred inner chalice, than ever, now.

Even as I share my story with you today, I feel a renewed surge of energy pulsing through my veins, anointing me with renewed fervor for guiding others through this same journey for themselves.

I am over-the-moon and beyond grateful for that fateful moment sitting on that swing where my Inner Goddess Guided me into a Life Re-imagined.

I am worthy, sacred, whole, and wholly consecrated in my body. I am home. I remember.

Reflection

What rituals exist within your family and are they ones you want to keep?

_____

_____

_____

_____

How have you judged your experiences compared to your peers?

_____

_____

_____

_____

In what ways have you embraced or rejected your body?

_____

_____

_____

_____

CHAPTER THREE

RELATIONSHIPS
Reimagined

Breaking My Vows, Healing My Heart

DR. DEBRA L. REBLE

*S*itting on the wobbly first step of my back deck on a cold spring day in March, I thought, "I can't do this to myself or my children any longer."

It felt like my feet were on the ground anchoring me in my current life while the rest of me was spinning out of control into my future. At the same time, I felt depressed and stuck. I had long been unhappy but had not allowed myself to feel the depth of my pain or to make an alternative choice. Yet I knew I was compromising myself by continuing to play the role of caretaker, keeping everything together to make others happy.

For over nine years, I felt as if I had been in emotional and spiritual limbo, going through the motions in my second marriage while setting my own needs aside for others. I knew this place well, for I had lived here all my life: waiting for the other shoe to drop, waiting for things to get better, and waiting for the courage to make a choice. I clung to my daily routines as a buoy so as not to slip into the sea of despair that threatened to engulf me. I knew I needed to lean into my pain and let it open me, but I was too afraid to do so. I also knew that in choosing to make my husband's life wonderful, I had temporarily forfeited my own fulfillment, along with my dream of genuine love and connection between myself and a true partner.

Lying on my bed, I was transported back to my living room on the night of my second husband's doctoral graduation party. I saw him standing, wearing a paper king's crown, and beaming triumphantly as friends and family congratulated him on his accomplishment. I watched from the shadows—not as his queen, but as a servant to his dreams, as always.

I had deferred my life for his in yet another self-sacrificial relationship. I had supported his dreams without asking for support of my own. In fact, trying to fix the relationship made me feel worthwhile and in control. I had created a familiar scenario—anticipating that a relationship would complete me—but instead of bringing us closer, our patterns of behavior had led to a situation where we led parallel but separate lives linked only through children and the house.

Even with my unrelenting love and support, he resisted doing his own spiritual work. He was content with his dependence on me and the stagnant day-to-day comfort zone of our relationship. In this graveyard of a marriage, trust, integrity, and intimacy were long gone; in their place grew a destructive kudzu vine of indifference that suppressed even discontent. I was living in passive coexistence of apathy and codependence.

From the perspective of my friends and family, my life appeared ideal. They saw a comfortable home, two well-adjusted children, and a marriage absent of external conflict. But what they observed was a facade. I tried to make my marriage work by taking care of everything, a deception that was encouraged by family and friends. They supported me as long as I tried to keep the relationship alive even when it had already spiritually died. Instead of listening to my own heart, I deferred to everyone else and their idea of what was best for me. Afraid of disappointing them, I had avoided the choice to leave my marriage, a choice I knew my heart had already made years ago.

Even though I knew in my heart that my marriage was over, I had tried to stick it out for my teenage son's benefit. I had already put him through the trauma of one divorce, and my heart couldn't bear to put him through another. I was terrified of breaking his heart, but most of all his spirit. Tom was only two years old when his father and I divorced. If I chose divorce again while he was sixteen, he would experience the break-up of his family, feel the devastating pain of loss, and go through the upheaval that a divorce brings with it.

My young daughter, however, was witnessing my role as a caretaker in a codependent relationship ... a relationship void of mutual responsibility and personal growth. Did I really want this to be her model for future relationships? I felt as if I was in a no- win situation. What would I say to my children who depended on me? How could I tell them in a way that wasn't devastating? Any choice I made—even if it was the choice to do nothing and change nothing—would end up hurting someone.

Because I had hidden my despair, Tom was shocked when I told him I was divorcing his stepfather. Even though I reassured him that he would stay in the same house and go to the same school, I knew he was devastated. There was nothing I could do to take away the pain that spoke to me through his eyes; yet I knew on a divine level that this was our journey together and that he would be okay. All I could do was trust myself and breathe love into him.

Having been told by her father that her parents would never get divorced, Alex fell apart in my arms the day I told her. So, I picked her up, drew a warm bath, and held her tightly in our deep clawfoot tub until her sobs stilled. All I could do was reassure her that she was loved and that it had nothing to do with her.

This was one of the hardest days of my life. I needed to share my paralyzing fear of repeating my legacy of divorce, so I called my brother. Shaken by shame about the failure of my marriage and anguish over putting my children through this kind of ordeal, I opened my heart and shared my vulnerability with him.

As I spoke, I experienced a flashback to the day I was told of my own parents' impending divorce. My heart had imprinted the emotional pain of this past trauma, and it was now surfacing through my entire body like superheated water erupting from a geyser. At that moment, I realized that I was superimposing my own experience on my children. I felt that I was putting them through the same difficult experience—the experience that had haunted me for so many years. But as I talked through the connection between this past pain and my present situation, I realized, I wasn't my mother, and my children weren't me. We were going to be okay because I only wanted the best for everyone involved. Exposing my deep pain and feeling supported through my vulnerability encouraged me to find self-compassion in the days to follow, even when things got emotionally intense. It also elevated my spiritual perspective and helped me see that my path was, in fact, my own.

The path wasn't without its rough patches. I had recently left my position as a school psychologist to become an entrepreneur in private practice. I had to refinance my house and buy out my ex-husband's equity in order to keep my children in their family home. But even though I had just left my steady job and had piles of debt from the marriage, the refinance went through on angel's wings. It felt like a sign from the Universe that I was being supported.

Before I could finally make the courageous choice to leave my marriage, I had to first forgive the vow I had made to myself that I would never put my children through this kind of experience. My heart was congested with feelings of disappointment, shame, and guilt for betraying them. Slowly, trusting myself and leaning into these layers, I sat with my pain instead of escaping from it into more distraction. I set aside time every day for meditation and journaling and faced my feelings "heart on" until they released. The more I released my feelings, the more I began to forgive myself for staying too long in another dysfunctional relationship. I realized I had made the best choices possible at the time. Trusting myself and letting go, I finally left my marriage—a choice that originated from the intention my brave heart had made that early spring day on my deck steps.

To create the space for a genuine, loving, and connected relationship, I had to let go of the relationship I was in and release the toxic residue left in its wake. Even though I was terrified of being divorced and single again, I knew on some level that I was inviting in an intense period of self-discovery and healing. Because I had always defined myself by my roles as a wife, mother, and caretaker, I felt untethered and uncertain, and questioned who I was and what I truly wanted. In letting go of my anger at myself and my ex-husband and forgiving the underlying disappointing loss of our relationship, I started to come out of the shadows of shame. I let my tears wash away a lifetime of unhealed loss. Like a cosmic cow catcher in front of a locomotive, I had to clear the track of anything that blocked the flow of love in my life. If I wanted to live a life of authenticity, I had to affirm that I was lovable and didn't need anyone's permission to be or express this love. And that, in turn, meant changing everything I knew about how to be in a loving and connected relationship.

The pivotal moment of inviting in real love and connection came when I found the courage to let go of my second marriage and chose to love myself more than the codependent patterns that had held my relationship together.

Reflection

What are your long-standing patterns of behavior in relationships? Do these patterns serve your happiness and well-being?

_____

_____

_____

_____

Whose well-being do you consider first in making important decisions? How do you balance your vows and obligations to others with the vows you've made to yourself?

_____

_____

_____

_____

What steps can you take to break free from old, unhelpful patterns and create the space for something new?

_____

_____

_____

_____

Finding the Way Home

NANCY OKEEFE

Sadness and grief had replaced the love, fun, and companionship my partner and I had. Bickering when we were together resulted in us keeping to separate corners of our home. We'd gone from lovers to roommates, and I couldn't see the way back. How had it happened? I tried to retrace my steps but couldn't. I was lost in the forest of unhappiness in a relationship that was falling apart. I felt panicky at the notion of what would happen if we didn't figure out how to fix things. No matter what I did or how much we talked it out nothing changed. He wasn't happy with me, and I wasn't happy with him. The fun loving, up-for-any-adventure, party-in-a box-guy I fell in love with had disappeared. I lived in a loveless relationship; the worst kind of loneliness of all.

Five years earlier, he suffered from a serious fall at work that caused major injury to his back. He fell and landed on a large beam with a second one falling on top of him. A year of countless treatments and back surgery left him with a lingering disability and constant back pain. I nurtured him, cared for him, and loved him through every treatment, even putting my business on hold for the first eight weeks after his surgery. His physical wounds healed, but the mental toll of never being able to work again, the loss of his identity after working in his field for thirty years, and the feeling that he no longer had value, took an emotional toll on both of us.

I was filled with sadness. The thirteen years before his accident had been some of the best in my life. "I can handle this" I told myself, "I'm strong." I repeatedly reminded myself, "It isn't his fault. He can't help it." I pushed my feelings down and tried to make every day as good as possible.

Most nights he was in bed by 7:30 p.m., and I used my alone time in front of the television to cry over the events of the day. Little by little, my sadness turned to resentment, and the resentment leaked out into our day, further straining our relationship. I felt angry. People suggested counseling but I couldn't bring myself to ask him to go. His physical situation wasn't going to change, and I didn't see how his attitude could change either. We were in a downward spiral neither one of us knew how to stop. Every night, I prayed for help. I prayed for an answer. I prayed for him. I prayed for me. I prayed for our relationship.

One day, I got an answer. It didn't come in the form of an idea or a thought or a voice. It came in a diagnosis. I had cancer.

Over the years, I studied a variety of energy healing modalities and, although I don't work in this area, I am an intuitive energy healer. I suddenly realized I had not tapped into what I know to be true: while nurturing and loving him, I'd ignored giving myself the same level of care. When negative energy gets stuck in the body, it can cause dis-ease. There it was, just as I had been taught. Cancer.

It took me a few days to come to grips with the diagnosis. Cancer was such a scary prospect. Having it was bad enough, but the stories about treatment were almost scarier than the dis-ease. I had friends who had chemotherapy, so I knew about the side effects. Suddenly, I needed him. But I worried that he wouldn't be able to be there for me. I worried about who was going to take care of me as I went through treatment. I worried that I would lose my hair. I worried that cancer might be the final blow to our relationship.

I had no choice but to look to him for help. I leaned on him, and he let me. We talked. We hugged. We cried.

Over the weeks before my treatment, we talked about our fears. He was concerned about meals and other things I routinely did for us that he knew nothing about. He didn't like to cook so we worked together to make up a dozen pre-cooked meals for the freezer that he could microwave during the first few weeks after my surgery. We cleaned the house and got everything as ready as we could, working together with the goal of making things as easy for both of us as possible.

All of a sudden, I realized something: there he was. The man I fell in love with. My protector, my lover, my friend. I watched him step up and lovingly do everything I needed despite his pain. I needed him and he needed to be needed. I allowed myself to be vulnerable and he took care of me.

During those first weeks, he did all of the chores. He made my meals. He helped me in and out of bed. If I dropped something, he rushed to pick it up. He fluffed my pillows. Rubbed my back. We talked, and realized we needed each other in ways we had not expressed in many years.

Fortunately, my cancer had a swift and successful conclusion. No other treatment was needed after the surgery. I felt lucky and deeply grateful. In my gratitude, I realized cancer had been given to me as a gift in answer to many nights of prayers. Cancer helped me get my life back on track and focus on the self-care I deserved. It helped me get my relationship back. It was the earth-shattering catalyst our relationship needed. It blew an opening in our situation like dynamite in a mineshaft. Light poured into the darkness and the way back to each other became clear.

Now we lovingly spend time every day together, enjoying each other's company. We have dreams again and are making plans to expand an outdoor living area for entertaining. We worked out a flexible plan that gives us time together in the morning with our afternoons for him resting and me work-ing. There is more balance and flow in life, and I feel more energized. The 7:30 p.m. bedtime has become the exception, not the norm. We even took a chair Yoga fitness class together. Life became easy and enjoyable. The bicker-ing stopped. The resentment vanished. We found our way back to more love and more laughter. We found our way home.

I think about this experience every day. I express my gratitude each night in my prayers, thanking the Universe that my dis-ease resolved so quickly and easily. But more importantly, I am left with the knowledge that I was given not one, but two glorious gifts: cancer and the realization that cancer was the answer to my prayers.

I will never again look at any situation in my life the same way. I know there are no coincidences in life. I know the Universe is supporting me. I know I am connected, heard, and my prayers answered. I know that no mat-ter what form the answer takes, I will always ask myself, "What is the gift I have just been given?" And I will forever embrace each gift as a catalyst for a life reimagined.

Reflection

What challenges in your life may have been given to you as a gift?

_____

_____

_____

_____

How does seeing your challenges as a gift change your perspective?

_____

_____

_____

_____

What will you do differently because of the gifts you have been given?

_____

_____

_____

_____

Nowhere to Go but Up

CHRISTIN BJERGBAKKE

Crying at the beach is really not to be recommended. This thought crossed my mind as I wiped away the tears, for the hundredth time, that were escaping the sheltered space behind my dark sunglasses. The sand on my fingers scratched my skin and inevitably got into my eyes, making me cry even harder. It wasn't fair. Life just wasn't fair.

I gave up reading my book, turned, and lay flat on my back. The emotional pain in my body was on a high frequency, slicing through my consciousness like a butcher's knife; the open wound blocking out anything else—a sharp white pain of panic, sorrow, and confusion all at the same time.

The tears filled my eyes, drop by drop, until I rose and went for a swim. Being held and embraced by Mother Ocean felt safe and comforting, allowing my tears to flow freely. Even so, the murmuring pain deep in my stomach and the heavy feeling of despair in my chest reminded me that things were not okay, and that I had no idea how to solve my problems. *Where would we live? How would I be able to support my children? Why was this happening to me again?*

My partner and I had just returned from our summer holiday with our three girls, my twin daughters and his youngest child. There had been talks prior to the holiday. He was bored in our relationship. We had both agreed to make an effort over the summer. Upon our return, with the girls continuing on to their other parents, he told me of his final decision to end our nine-year long relationship. I was in shock! Panic and disbelief hit me hard. At the same time, I somehow knew deep down, that this was for the best. I was just so scared of how to handle it, that I could hardly breathe.

Having returned from a bank meeting where I was denied a house loan, reality hit me while I poured some wine, that I desperately thought I needed. Out of despair I had slid down onto the floor and hadn't been able to move since, feeling completely lost and powerless. Suppressed emotions built up over many years came flooding out, "How come these things keep happening to me? Why did I allow yet another man to have so much control over my life that I have no idea what to do when he cuts me loose? This cannot be the truth about me, this is not who I am!"

I cried out loud to Spirit, "This is it guys, I need you to step in and show me what the talk is all about." Right in that moment, I knew things had to change. I had to stop being a victim in my own life and blaming others for my misfortune.

Ten years earlier, the father of my children had left me for another woman. We had had some difficult years with mental illness and financial instability, but I stayed put out of fear of becoming a single mum and in the hope that we could rediscover our love. When his affair with a mutual friend was revealed, I was in shock. I didn't see it coming then, just as I hadn't seen it coming now. A pattern was repeating itself. My partner was the bad guy and I the innocent victim waiting for love to return. At least that's what I tried to convince myself: I was completely innocent and unaware of how bad things had actually grown between us. But this wasn't really the truth.

Reality was, that for quite a while my partner and I had been slipping apart. I had tried to talk to him about it, but he refused to admit anything was going on. You know, the mysterious text messages, sudden meetings in other parts of the country that required nights in hotels, excuses from him to avoid being intimate in the bedroom. I ignored it because I was afraid of the consequences if I didn't. For some years, he had been supporting me and my daughters, allowing me to pursue my dream of changing career path. Business was not booming, and I struggled to create a decent income in my new profession. In this process, I had let go of the responsibility of my own finances and placed the power over my family into the hands of another person, convincing myself that I couldn't make it on my own.

The growing imbalance between us resulted in him becoming more dominant and aggressive and me gaining weight and losing my mojo. We had come so off balance in our relationship, and I accepted it out of low self-esteem and misplaced gratitude, doubting my ability to create the life of my dreams. When the break-up became a reality, I had to find a way to support my daughters and be the best mum possible to my sweet girls.

Simply getting up from the kitchen floor that evening was my turning point. It wasn't like a strike of lightning and suddenly I knew all the answers, more like a lot of hard work. Over the next weeks, I slowly embraced the

Divine possibility of change. I had always believed that things happened for a reason. I now stopped looking for this reason elsewhere and started looking at my own actions. I realized that for most of my life I had given away my power out of fear, made myself dependent on others, and blamed the circumstances when things went wrong. Instead of staying victimized and helpless, I now managed to move myself to a place of power and hope. From here I was able to activate the tools I already knew from my work as a spiritual coach. Meditation to calm my nervous system, Reiki self-practice during the long nights, essential oils to lift my emotions, and daily talks with Spirit, "I place my trust in You, show me the next step."

I realized I had to do things differently, swallowed my pride and asked for help within my network. Not begging to be saved but asking for assistance. Saying out loud that I needed help was a big step for me and it was rewarded accordingly. One morning the oracle cards said, "Expect a Miracle." Reading it, I felt a tiny butterfly of hope unfold its wings from inside my stomach. The next day I received financial support presented as a gift from my parents that made it possible for me to rent a small house. This was indeed a miracle since my father had lost his business some years before and had been ill ever since. I had the weirdest feeling that Spirit had twisted some turns to make this possible. I started to follow every sign and nudge from Above. Transitioning from a lifelong superstition of not being worthy of making money to a place of complete trust. My daily affirmation became, "I am blessed, I am protected, I have all my wishes and desires fulfilled by the Universe."

This shift in my belief system was a complete game changer. I found my inner voice and began communicating from my heart. I developed skills I never thought would be within my reach and as if by magic new clients were attracted to me. My business is now thriving with an international clientele, we have a beautiful home, and my daughters are attending college on scholarships. I am no longer a victim stuck in my own limited beliefs and I wake up happy and grateful every morning. When I started listening to Spirit and acted accordingly my life was reinvented. I live in complete trust that I am supported by the Divine as long as I stay true to my heart. The minute I slide back into fear, Spirit gently shows me that I need to realign.

I am now aware that it is safe to create the life of my dreams by simply being me. By following the wisdom of my soul, I am no longer that victim crying at the beach.

Reflection

How has receiving a "no" turned out to be a blessing?

_____

_____

_____

_____

What relationship patterns have repeated in your life and what can you learn about yourself from them?

_____

_____

_____

_____

Where in your life have you asked for and received a miracle? What was the impact?

_____

_____

_____

_____

Learning to Love Myself

KIM BROCHU

*O*ne warm Texas evening in the spring of 2003, I drove home from a Mary Kay meeting, listening to Christina Aguilera's song *Beautiful,* roar from the speakers. As I sang along, a lump formed in my throat. The heavy, humid air hung in the car and I suddenly felt my chest and stomach tighten. Sadness flooded through me. I pulled off the road and burst into tears. Christina's words conflicted with my inner most thoughts. My marriage was falling apart, I certainly didn't feel beautiful, and I didn't know how to love myself. I dried my tears then pulled back onto the road for the short trip home, stuffing my emotions as far down as I could.

"I am not," I replied angrily to my best friend a few days later when she gently and lovingly suggested I was in denial about my marriage. Later, as I sat alone in my room, I considered her comment.

I thought back to all the phone calls he took quietly in the bathroom, how he worked longer hours, and how I was never able to reach him unless he called me.

The signs were clear, but I chose to push my feelings deep down and go on with my daily routine, instead of heeding them. It was easier just to ignore the red flags and believe every lie he offered up. But deep inside, it felt like a storm was barreling my way and that I couldn't shelter us if it hit. I'd convinced myself that if I ignored the obvious, the life shattering tornado would shift course, spare us, and everything would be fine.

Fear of the truth paralyzed me. Fear of what I thought was my worst nightmare coming true held me captive until I had nowhere else to hide.

And then the storm hit.

It's true what they say, about things getting worse before they get better. Over the next couple of months, I lost my husband when he announced he was leaving us, I lost my father to cancer, I lost my home, my car, and most of what I owned.

I found myself on a train traveling 1,700 miles back to our family, my three children all under the age of twelve in tow, one suitcase for each of us.

"I'll come soon, and we can work all of this out" my husband said.

I clung to his words as if they were the air I needed to breathe. Believing him gave me the strength to not grab my kids, run across the platform, and jump back into the car.

Instead, he got off the train after getting us settled, returned to his car, and drove away before we pulled out of the station.

There were times that my children and I lived in a run-down apartment that reeked of cat pee, and I don't know how I managed to feed us. Every time I tried to eat, my stomach rejected food. I laid in bed, willing myself to get up to take care of my kids when all I wanted to do was drink myself to sleep. I wanted to wake up from the nightmare our lives had become and find out none of it had really happened. I knew my children needed me, but I felt as if I was only half alive.

I felt frightened and incapable of helping myself, let alone them.

Fast forward several months, after another move, a bout of bronchitis, a dangerously rapid fifty-pound loss of weight, a habitual dependence on alcohol—and I found myself asking, *can I really go on?*

And then one morning, with my daughters at school and my son in daycare, I sat drowning in my own darkness and poured my first drink of the day. With each numbing gulp, I thought, *how can I go on? I can't raise my three children alone. I haven't worked in years. We have no money, we're on welfare, and I don't know how to pull myself up from here. It would be so much easier to just give up.*

I sat at the tiny, hand-me-down table we'd been given, and I prayed, my head on my hands, weary, shaking, and broken.

I can't be sure what gave me the strength to do what I did next—call it God, the Universe, Spirit—it doesn't matter. I thought of my children, and I picked up the phone.

I called therapists, leaving voicemail messages for them because their offices were not open that early. I begged them to call me back, telling them I didn't think I could make it through another day.

And then I welcomed the numbness as I continued to self-medicate, until finally someone called me back. Over the next week, I showed up at the therapist's office every day, as it was the only way she could justify not recommending inpatient care, diagnosing me with depression, anxiety, and suicidal thoughts. She accommodated my need to care for my kids because they needed me, and I could not fail them. I wanted help! I wanted to heal!

Life didn't improve immediately. As a matter of fact, it was a very long, very difficult road for all of us. What changed was some part of me nudging me to look within, to confront my negative ways, my old beliefs and fears, and to trust that we'd be okay.

I drifted off-course many times, sometimes willingly—almost defiantly, because doing the personal growth work was exhausting! *Why did I have to work so hard to heal and change?* Slowly, step by step, my kids and I picked ourselves up and moved on.

I had opened the door of possibility; allowed myself to believe that I could actually heal, that a better life was ahead of us; and with each baby step I took, more doors flew open.

I learned EFT, began to meditate, discovered karmic astrology, and I continued to pray and trust that I was supported, guided, and loved. I learned about healing the inner child and how to connect with her. New friends and mentors came into my life, people that propelled and supported my journey. But it wasn't until my self-sabotaging ways and worst fears, surfaced and came to light, that I could accept that there was no one else that could do my inner work for me, but me. It was time to love myself.

And now I'm the one answering the phone to hear a woman on the other end who is in a dark place and ready to heal. This is why I share my story, as difficult as it is at times, so that women will know they're not alone.

I sometimes wonder, did I show my kids that we can rise from the darkest places in life, or do they just see my failures?

Will they see the strength we all hold within us, rather than the weakness I once embraced? I can only hope so. Would I change any of it? I want to scream "yes" I would! But my soul quietly whispers "no" that I wouldn't change any of it because who I am today, and what our lives have become, is beyond anything I could have ever imagined.

Reflection

Have you ever found yourself at a point when you felt you could not go on, and how did you handle it?

_____

_____

_____

_____

Can you recall a moment when you were grateful that you reached out for help?

_____

_____

_____

_____

At a low point in your life, what or who motivated you to go on?

_____

_____

_____

_____

Reigniting My Spark

ANGELA SHAKTI SPARKS

"I'm not happy. I think we need some time apart," my husband solemnly told me.

My heart sank as I realized I might lose the only good thing in my life. My body constricted as a wave of pain surged through me, tears welling up in my eyes. I certainly didn't blame him. I knew I wasn't emotionally available, and I'd spent the previous year slipping into a deep depression, lying on the floor nearly every day, Elizabeth Gilbert *Eat, Pray, Love*-style, begging for someone to help me. I was a mess.

In fact, much of my life could be summed up as a big hot mess, with intense emotional suffering, unending health problems, recurring bouts of depression, and a pattern of unhealthy relationships. Life was an emotional roller coaster with more lows than highs and I often felt like a victim of life's circumstances in a cruel and unforgiving world.

As a little girl, I frequently suffered from migraines, incessant throat infections, and terrible nightmares. With each passing year, my playful, curious, imaginative nature was dampened as I took on the weight of the world, being highly sensitive to the emotions and energies of those around me.

In my teens, I turned to drugs and alcohol in an attempt to numb the pain and escape the hypocrisy I saw all around me. Then, at sixteen, the death of my boyfriend in a car accident gave me my first taste of blinding grief. My rebellion and anger at the world doubled in intensity.

A verbally abusive high school relationship followed and made me feel utterly worthless. I came close to taking my life, holding a handful of pills as I wrestled with thoughts of ending it all.

In college, I reveled in my newfound freedom and indulged my passions for dance and travel. However, I stayed fickle in my relationships, fortifying the wall around my heart to keep only surface-level commitments.

Just out of college, I married my first husband, which was my healthiest relationship to date. Yet seven years in, I couldn't ignore my nagging discontent. With different visions for our futures and a lack of communication, we eventually divorced.

I soon began dating my current husband who had also left a long-term relationship. We had a magnetic connection and married a year later. We had a passionate physical attraction and a mutual love of social activities with friends and family.

However, the honeymoon was over all too soon. I was reactive and easily hurt, having brought my hidden fears of loss and abandonment, need for external validation, and a ton of emotional baggage along for the ride.

All the emotions I'd been suppressing throughout my life ate away at me. My muscles were in constant pain and the traditional medical system continued to fail me in finding an answer. The physical and emotional pain became unbearable to the point where I sobbed daily, and some days couldn't muster the energy to get out of bed.

Looking back, I'm surprised we lasted as long as we did before my husband lost hope in us. I was devastated at the thought of losing him but agreed to take some time apart. It felt as though I'd fallen to the bottom of a deep abyss with no way out.

I went to my sister's house, spending the next week locked away in a bedroom, sobbing. It was as if I cried for all of the pain I'd been numbing and avoiding all my life, but was being forced to face.

I eventually cried myself into utter exhaustion. In that moment, as I lay raw, bare, and open, I suddenly realized that no matter how much I cried, begged, and prayed, nothing outside of me was going to save me. Not the medical community, a parent, friend, or any partner. If anything was going to change, it was up to me.

Up to that point, I'd been under the erratic rule of my emotions and victimhood consciousness, with the stories and patterns of my past dictating my present. But a powerful determination swelled within me to turn my life around, climb out of that abyss, and, if at all possible, save my marriage.

A fervent search ensued for alternative solutions for my depression and health issues and I approached conversations with my husband as calmly as possible. Serendipitously, a book about empaths found its way to me and instantly so much of my life made sense. Memories of events throughout my life replayed in my mind as I read how empaths literally feel the emotions of others, are hypersensitive, are prone to chronic health conditions and depression, and can have difficulty maintaining healthy relationships.

Aha! I wasn't just a big hot mess after all but was rather an unaware empath taking on the energy of the world as if it were my own and navigating the best I could. Learning this about myself gave me immense hope. I finally felt I had the missing piece to all my pain and suffering.

Exploring various holistic practices, I cleared layer after layer of buried emotions, resolving past traumas, and nurturing my wounded inner child. I tapped, journaled, danced, and worked with energy medicine and soul retrieval. I discovered Ayurveda and began seeing a holistic doctor. Yoga and meditation practices reignited my deeply spiritual nature and reconnected me with Divine Source.

Surprisingly, the inner work wasn't nearly as difficult as I thought it would be. I rather enjoyed all that I was learning, and I never could have imagined how light and freeing it would feel! My physical health improved, I saw more possibility, and I discovered that many of the emotions I'd been carrying weren't even mine.

All of my relationships improved in the process. I became less reactive, more emotionally balanced, and learned to strengthen my energetic and personal boundaries. In breaking through the wall I'd built around my heart, I cultivated forgiveness and compassion for myself and others, opening the way for deeper connection and joy.

My husband and I slowly rebuilt our relationship and are now happier than we ever imagined was possible. It was a bumpy road at times, yet as I focused on healing my maladaptive patterns rather than trying to get him to change, we experienced ever improving communication and connection. This involved the on-going practice of standing in my truth and surrendering to the possibility that, in doing so, I might lose him. It was scary and wasn't easy, yet absolutely worth it. In a way, I feel that he respects me more because of it.

We also both continue to evolve and support each other in our growth. The emotional healing we embarked on, each in our own time, without being pressured, has allowed us to experience a deeper level of love, which wasn't possible when we kept our hearts guarded or were living our old stories.

I'm so grateful for the love we share and the love I am able to feel for others and for life. I am grateful my playfulness, creativity, and passion for life have been reignited. I appreciate my emotions as the exquisite guidance system they are, and I'm ever grateful for my health and true happiness. A life I once couldn't wait to end, I now desire to explore and enjoy deeply for decades to come!

Those of us who are empaths or highly sensitive often suffer profoundly and attract dysfunctional relationships. It is a gift, yet until we know how to work with it, it can feel like a curse. When we learn to tune into our emotional guidance system and let go of what isn't ours, we open the way for uplifting, joyful emotions to emerge. Not only are we uplifted, we uplift others and the world by holding higher vibrations. When we stand in our truth, honor our boundaries, have the courage to heal our past, and let our light shine, we inspire others to do the same…and in the process, we get to finally live a truly joyful, healthy, and fulfilling life. Yes, please, and thank you!

Reflection

How do you deal with unpleasant or painful emotions? If you are an empath or highly sensitive person, when you feel an unpleasant emotion, do you take a moment to discern if it is yours or someone else's?

_____

_____

_____

_____

What unhealthy patterns and old stories have you brought into your current or previous relationship? What steps can you take to dissolve these patterns?

_____

_____

_____

_____

Where are you not setting boundaries that honor and support your needs and authenticity? What is one boundary you can set this week?

_____

71

_____

_____

_____

The "What Next?" Woman

KIMMBERLY WOTIPKA

For as long as I could remember, I had wanted to be a lawyer. I was born at the beginning of Generation X, a time where women were told they could do anything they wanted—and didn't need a man to do it for them.

After I graduated from high school though, something shifted. I needed out of that small Texas town and away from everyone and everything associated with it. I thought the quickest and best way to do that was to get married.

Fast forward twenty years and three kids later—I wanted out again. All I could do at that point was grapple with the anonymity of the previous twenty years. I had always been someone's mother, wife, or daughter. My entire life had been about everyone else, and I didn't know who I was without them.

I started a marketing business that, with the help of child support, paid the bills for me and my three daughters, who were seventeen, fourteen, and eleven. We hobbled along for about three years. By that time, the oldest had left home and had a baby of her own. My middle daughter was headed to college in the fall and the youngest would stay with me.

I had taken my girls to San Diego for Spring Break the year before and done a few silent retreats at an Ashram Center there. I loved the area and beach life called me. I asked my youngest daughter to move there with me, and she said she would, albeit with some trepidation. I knew moving to a new place might be scary for her, but somehow, I believed she wanted to move as much as I did.

As I was buying the plane tickets, she told me she didn't want to leave her friends, had already talked with her dad, and would be staying in Illinois with him.

What…? I had built my life around my kids. How could she do that to me? How could she leave me? It took me a little more time to decide that I would go with or without her. I couldn't remain stuck anymore. I sold everything I owned and landed in Los Angeles that August on my birthday.

I fully intended to make a life for myself in California. A few months in though, and the pressure of being away from everything and everyone I had ever known, in addition to the pressure of dealing with so many clients for my marketing agency, began to take its toll. I craved some time to myself to figure out what I really wanted moving forward.

I attended a silent retreat in a neighboring town with beautiful gardens overlooking the ocean. My soul was wearied from all the struggles of the past and present and sorely needed restoration. I was fed up with feeling like a failure at everything I did.

Being there, I understood the quiet self-reflection that is born of complete silence. I felt like a huge weight had been lifted off my shoulders and the frenetic energy of everyday life had disappeared. I felt ready to take on life again, but I never wanted to leave!

And yet I did, and after that place, I experienced what I would later refer to as a "dark night of the soul." My dark *night* lasted a solid month. That entire month of October was spent barely moving from my bed. The despair of having left it all behind, yet not knowing what was ahead, was crippling. It was the most difficult, yet significant time of my life.

Over the Thanksgiving holiday, my ex-husband remarried, and they wanted both his and her kids to be there. I was living in a friend's studio with no car, few friends, and nothing of my own. So, I headed to Texas to be with my family for the holidays.

I had also met someone online that lived in the same area as my parents and that was a welcome diversion. Although I could not see it at the time, I was looking for another rescue. However, he expected me to return to California and I hadn't even booked a return ticket—fully believing that he and I would hit it off and he would ask me to stay.

I stopped pushing that relationship after a couple of weeks and gave up. I was resigned to the fact that I was an utter and complete failure in every aspect; as a wife, a mother, and a woman who wanted to make it on her own but never really knew how.

After Christmas, my parents realized how much I was struggling, and they offered me a place to stay with them for as long as I wanted. It felt so good to have them want me there! My youth was mostly spent in rebellion, so having this time with them was like getting a do-over.

Living with my parents wasn't exactly smooth sailing. I didn't want to juggle clients anymore but struggled to find a job after being self-employed for so long. It was also difficult to live in another woman's house when I was used to running my own, even if the other woman was my mother.

Eventually, life came together. I realized that if I was going to be alone and make it on my own, I needed to take better care of myself emotionally and physically. I set better boundaries with my children and family. I practiced saying "No" a lot! I just didn't have the energy or brain space for certain things anymore. I stopped trying to please everyone and stopped trying to do everything by myself. I had to let go of quite a bit of resentment and anger about my childhood. Having that time with my parents was helpful for that. Most importantly, I forgave myself for even getting to the point of feeling like a failure and struggling in the first place.

At the beginning of the summer, I found a job with a healthcare company as a project manager and was finally able to buy a car. I got serious about learning how to consciously create a radiant life for myself and was dreaming big for the first time in my life.

Creating this movement in my life with the job and car and taking care of myself helped me to stop feeling like a victim, to stop being afraid, and to stop feeling hopeless and powerless. I had searched for the place where I belonged for so long; constantly seeking that place outside of myself had been exhausting. But when I realized it had been within me all along, is when my life completely changed.

I was surprised to run into an old friend in town one evening. She asked me to meet her at her brother's house for a glass of wine. The minute I walked through that door, I sensed that it was the door I was meant to walk through my whole life. Six weeks later, we went to Vegas and he proposed. We were married just three months after that. It was just like getting another amazing do-over in life—first with my parents, and then with my first real crush. And it was glorious to not have to be anyone—but ME!

That was almost nine years ago, and I am so grateful every day that I have this amazing life, that I could not have ever imagined I would have before.

Many of us never receive reassurance, that no matter how horrible life gets, we will eventually, not just be okay, but thrive. When I began a practice of connecting to the place within that has never been afraid, I felt a grounded presence that made me sure and confident and peaceful all at once. I'd love to be able to hug that earlier version of me and tell her, "It's all going to work out. Everything is okay. You are loved."

From every single one of our "What Next?" moments comes transformation. We dig deep, see fear for the inhibitor it is, and take action. My terrifying What Next moments have given me profound experiences of feeling excited, creative, happy, appreciated, and as if I am making a difference in the world. Every day, I experience my inner radiance—the part of me that has always been there. The part of me that feels like a Radiant Queen.

Reflection

Can you recall a time when you felt stuck? How did you handle it?

_____

_____

_____

_____

When you feel stuck, what prompts you to take action?

_____

_____

_____

_____

Write about a time when you felt sure of making a big and scary decision.

_____

_____

_____

_____

CHAPTER FOUR

SPIRIT
Reimagined

Ready or Not

CARA HOPE CLARK

From the beginning of our romance and throughout our eighteen years together, my husband Claude viewed me as a strong and powerful woman. Though I absolutely sensed that this was true, I was not yet able to fully embrace my personal power and my truest essence. Though limiting and frustrating, my faithful cloaking device used by the shy, highly sensitive little girl inside served its purpose. I contentedly stayed safely tucked away in the shadows. Even so, I did grow in many ways over the years as we created our life together. Still, Claude continued to lovingly nudge me in the direction of embodying more of those qualities we both knew I was capable of. But I wasn't ready.

Nevertheless, *ready or not*, in a blink of an eye, I was plunged into the deep end when my dear beloved husband took his own life in the sanctity our home. My unprepared heart was utterly shattered. In an instant, I became a widow, residing with our fourteen-year-old son in our unfathomable reality. I was left wondering, *who am I now without my other half, the man who I had devoted my heart and soul to?*

With the weight of my grief bearing down on me and our lives forever altered, there was no longer any room to play it small. Without a doubt, new aspects of me as a strong and powerful woman were activated during this time. I had to find a way to keep moving forward, showing up to raise my son, managing a multitude of personal estate issues, selling a business, properties, his car, and motorcycle, plus eventually moving to another state. All while caught in the maze of unyielding trauma and grief.

As a former massage therapist and energetic healer, I knew the importance of reaching out for support. Over time, I assembled a team of varied practitioners who held my hand as I moved through this unimaginable time. I slowly healed my heart, and, in the process, evolved in innumerable ways, specifically learning how to step more into my masculine energies to manage the varied responsibilities thrust upon me. Working with my healers, I accessed more of my feminine intuition. I became a more conscious and balanced human.

I still hid in many ways due to the nature of grief. Yet, I slowly emerged from my chrysalis. With the persistent and purposeful inner work

I had done, my True Self blossomed and came to the forefront in new ways. Though I had always been an intuitive empath and quite used to following my inner knowing, new insights were being fully activated during this time.

Two years after Claude's suicide, my son Noah and I moved to Boulder, Colorado to make a fresh start. Soon after, I began hearing the whispers from my angelic guides, *"We want you to share your story of healing and transformation after Claude's suicide; you will help many. We want you to write a book!"*

I thought, *What? I am not a writer! I was a disaster in English!* I responded point blank, *"If you want me to write this book, you need to give me the words and the guidance on how to make it happen."*

They assured me that the path was already laid out and that I simply needed to show up to bring the book into form. It sounded simple enough, but I wasn't ready, yet.

The limiting beliefs and outdated programs operating within my being still ran the show. I felt frightened to put myself in the public eye, scared of being judged, of being seen, afraid that I wouldn't do the story justice, and vulnerable about bringing my life's most horrific event to print.

Despite this hesitation, I felt an aching deep in my soul that this was truly my path. I tapped into even more of my personal power by designing and setting up a website with the intention of writing a blog around grief support. Over that two-year period, much to my amazement, I discovered my voice as a writer. Eventually, I signed up for an online course where I learned how to write my memoir.

Though in many ways the creative process enlivened me, after spending several months immersed in writing my first draft, it also deeply strained me emotionally and physically. Sharing my truth required reliving the past again and again. Plus, the realization of the overwhelming prospect of how to publish and promote my book, the cost involved…it all felt daunting. I questioned my commitment to this project and put it aside.

Looking back, I see that I let my fears and doubt get back into the driver's seat, steering me off course. Though I gave into this protective mechanism, clearly fashioned by my personality or small self, I often considered what my life would have looked like if I had stayed on track. *Would I always wonder what would have happened if I followed through to completion? Would regret be my unceasing companion?* After all, it seemed that writing my book was a divinely appointed mission that I had chosen to abort.

It took almost two years to surmount that presumed fall from grace. I woke up one unremarkable December morning to my angels gently tapping me on the shoulder again. I was in the bathroom getting ready for my day when suddenly I received the clear message: *Why not contact an editor to see if what you have written so far in your book might be worth finishing?* It was a subtle yet powerful voice that I chose *not* to ignore.

Listening and trusting this divine inspiration was one of the most pivotal choices that I have ever made. Was I still scared? Yup! But after sending my first draft to an editor and receiving an editorial review about a month later, I was all in! The time had come to go for it.

In hindsight, unknowingly taking a sabbatical was actually by divine purpose. I had evolved during that respite. As a result, I was able to transmit a deeper exploration of my transformational journey, infusing my memoir with more wisdom than I would have brought previously.

I didn't know at the onset that my book writing process would be one of the most empowering experiences of my life. Was it hard and challenging? Yes! Did I consider quitting again? Not on your life! Writing my story surely tested my strength and felt grueling at times, as if I were running a marathon against myself. But it also felt incredibly freeing, with the unexpected bonus of taming many of my fears. I could breathe a sigh of relief having fulfilled my soul's directive. I had climbed the insurmountable mountain knowing that Claude had kept his promise to figuratively hold my hand from the other side, supporting me as I moved through my fears and uncertainties.

In addition, much to my amazement, I learned over time that grief had become a gift from my soul, an unexpected teacher, a catalyst for growth and transformation. It wasn't at all clear at the onset of the nine-year cycle following Claude's suicide that I would steadily move in the direction of becoming that woman that we both had glimpses of years before.

My memoir was published in the summer of 2021, so the road before me is still fresh and new. Only time will tell where it will lead me. My heart is filled with gratitude that I said yes to healing, yes to writing and sharing my story, yes to showing up as the strong and powerful courageous woman who embraces her purposeful calling. As a sovereign co-creator, I trust that my path forward will be illuminated by one step and then the next. I am excited to see where my guides will lead me as I progress on this dynamic reimagined path filled with unlimited possibility.

Reflection

What has your heart been longing for? Are you allowing yourself the freedom to move forward with that dream or action?

_____

_____

_____

_____

Are you allowing your inner guidance to lead you to your soul's purpose? If not, what limiting beliefs can you acknowledge and shift to assist you in moving in the direction of your dreams?

_____

_____

_____

_____

What fears are holding you back from speaking your truth and shining your light in the world? What would your world look like if you were to step into the light of your soul?

_____

_____

_____

Nature's Way Open

AMBER KASIC

*H*ave you ever traced with your eyes the fall of a leaf through the autumn air, admiring the beauty, and wondering just how long the wind would carry it this way and that before it inevitably falls to its new home? Ten days before my dad's passing, we took a photo together under a gorgeous, full yellow maple tree. His life was soon ending, and I knew it. My hand rested on his heart as we stared into each other's eyes, silently recognizing a shared lifetime of a sometimes complicated father-daughter relationship. I smiled, burying the tears welled up in my heart. What was sometimes so complex was suddenly so simple. I just loved my perfectly imperfect dad.

During one of our last, mostly lucid, conversations I asked for an agreed-upon signal to know he was well in his new "home." I pushed through my nerves to be vulnerable and ask for what I wanted. Dad hadn't wanted to talk at all about dying.

"How about a leaf in my face, Dad?"

He grunted in disapproval of my suggestion, so I made two more, finally settling on a deer walking in my path, my dad adding, "Everything will be near. You'll know in the eyes."

"I don't know what exactly is possible, Dad, but I believe in possibilities," I said. I closed my eyes and laid back in the chair, thankful for having listened to my heart's nudge.

Days later, my dad entered the state of final transition and hadn't uttered a sound for twenty-four hours. It seemed unimaginable to never again hear his strong, yet soothing voice which, just days ago, had brought comfort to my heart as he sang me a few bars of a childhood song. Keeping vigil at his bedside, I remembered obsessing over the amount of suffering and fear he might endure in this time, causing a long emotional torment of my own. Whether exploring possible criminal consequences of giving my dad too much morphine in the end, or sleepless nights spent reading horoscopes and researching the death process, in a desperate attempt to know exactly when and how he would die, for two years I tried to be perfectly prepared for an event that, like birth, is its own miracle and can only be supported, not controlled.

Lying alongside Dad in his hospice bed, my head on his broad chest and his warm hand in mine, I surrendered myself to Nature's Way like a leaf to the wind just ripped from its tree. This journey was my dad's to take and I needed to learn to let him go. In that stillness, I detached from all the what-ifs, disappointments, and grief, and instead put my power in full presence and unconditional love.

In that moment of surrender, I experienced what I describe as *not of me*. As we lay peacefully, hands entwined, I suddenly witnessed hues of purple swirling in my mind's vision, and felt an incredible warmth encompass my entire body. I thought surely the sun from the window was playing tricks on me. But then with full clarity, I felt an energy enter my back, go into my heart center and swirl around, before moving to my shoulder, from which point I followed the feeling as it traveled slowly down my arm, into my hand, and, lastly, I just KNEW with total certainty, into my dad.

I hugged my dad tight and whispered in his ear, "Dad, I don't know what that was, but I hope you felt it too. Take all that love and light in your core with you and leave the old news behind." I knew, deep within my soul, my dad and I were eternally bonded. I never imagined it possible to feel such peace at such a painful time.

At 4:00 a.m. on November 1, with me curled beside him, his hand in mine, my dad took his final resting breath. I had accompanied him on his journey as far as God would allow.

Following my dad's death, I learned that, like the leaf that is no longer on the tree but remains in the world, my dad was not gone at all—not because I wished it to be so, but because his energy remained, and I could feel, hear, and sometimes even engage with his spirit.

The first true awareness I had was hearing his voice in my mind. Shortly after he died, I drove to a park for a walk but found myself too mentally exhausted to move.

"Get out of the car, Ambie. You've cried enough tears over me in your life," my dad said inside my head.

It was true. I had cried more tears in my life than a daughter ever should, but where had that voice come from? I did as he said, taking a path through tall pines. I said, "I hope you're alright, Dad."

Instantly, I heard him respond, "I'm fine, Ambie. I've got to stick around here a while and help some people, and I'm happy about it."

I stopped walking, stunned. *Surely, I'm making this up,* I thought, but I knew I didn't think that way. I would have said, "Heaven's so beautiful and I am with my parents and Granddad again. Our beloved dogs, Thunder and Bailey, are here and love you." Now curious, I wondered, *is it possible my dad is connecting with me somehow? And who would he be helping?*

I didn't trust this voice at first, but my otherworldly experiences with him grew, accompanied by information I could have never known, and signs and synchronicities without any other possible explanation. My dad now being the wind and me the leaf, shook me from my tree of logic, stability, and control, and during the next months, led me through a transformation toward my inner Light. One I have come to know we all possess, as beings of spirit having a human experience. This Light also simultaneously connects us all.

With this awareness of Light, I see with new eyes and feel with a new sense of being. What once was a pleasurable walk in the woods can now be experienced as a joyous state of union with life. Hanging Christmas decorations with family transformed from a fun seasonal activity to an experience of genuine joy and hope. I am learning to become aware of what arises within when I surrender to presence in my daily life, meditation, and relationships. Our Light is different from feelings of happiness. It's learning to experience the unwavering love, joy, and connection that is our soul.

In this place of pure rawness, I soon began to experience the Light of other souls from beyond the veil. From a colleague I barely knew, providing striking evidence and messages for his wife I never met, to an acquaintance's brother who died as a teenager with evidence and messages for his sister; to relatives of colleagues, I rarely spoke with; their Light arose in my awareness, and I surrendered to each experience.

In an especially touching moment, the father of a dear friend, who died during my friend's toddler years, and about whom I knew very little, extended his hand to me in my mind's eye, so as to shake it for an introduction, after having provided me with clear evidence and messages. And during

85

this reach of the hand, he said, with a smile and laugh at the humor of the situation, "Nice to finally meet you."

The magic of the wind carrying me on this journey has shown, through its whispers and visions, that we are not alone.

You are not alone.

We are supported in our lives even when it's unrecognizable to our hearts.

After six months, I have finally landed. My world was turned upside down, as I'm no longer a part of the tree and will never return. I hold the inner knowing that I am supported and, just where I am supposed to be, as I discover how my experiences will breathe new life into the world. I am in the place in between my own spiritual death and rebirth, and I know the path forward is found in the continued surrender to this beautiful life, and in the alignment with the Light that is me, you, and everything all at once. My dad was led home, and me open. Nature's Way is beautiful.

Reflection

In what ways might the practice of surrender benefit your own life?

_____

_____

_____

_____

In which of your personal relationships might attention to presence and unconditional love provide a benefit to your well-being?

_____

_____

_____

_____

What inner knowing, coming from your heart, do you possess about your life that might be helpful to trust?

_____

_____

_____

_____

Knowing Without Seeing

DONNA LABAR

I was in the medical center hallway phone booth in tears. It was November 24, 1998. My daughter had just been diagnosed with acute myeloid leukemia. Monica had been sick for weeks. She struggled through the start of seventh grade, feeling achy and tired every day. I thought her complaints stemmed from her being on the swim and cross-country teams. But a few weeks after the school year started, she was sent home with flu-like symptoms.

Convinced she had a virus, we followed up with the doctor. Weeks went by. She continued to be weak and dizzy with no appetite. Finally, we were sent to a medical center for an infectious disease team to see if they could determine the cause of her continued struggle. It wasn't long before oncology and hematology were also brought in. Then came the devastating diagnosis.

They gave her two weeks to live. *How could this be?* Her bone marrow was one hundred percent cancer. She was so ill that she slept most of the time. The team suggested I put her in a children's cancer study protocol to learn what they could from her case. Numb, with no time and limited choices, I sobbed as I signed for her to be part of a randomized treatment.

As she slept, I walked down the hall, trying to catch my breath and clear my mind. The next day, on my fortieth birthday, my beautiful child would begin chemotherapy. I stumbled upon some stylish wooden phone booths, complete with sliding doors, located at the end of a long hallway—a place that became a refuge for the next year. I went inside one and shut the door before allowing myself to crumble. I sobbed. The phone booth provided a sanctuary for me to fall apart in relative privacy before steeling myself to head back into the battle.

It was in that phone booth on the first day of Monica's treatment that I realized in my heart that she would not die. Prior to that moment of clarity, I'd been consumed by shock, panic, and sadness. That hope instantly gave me a profound thought.

Ten years earlier, my mother died from a massive heart attack. She was only fifty years old. I lost my mother at thirty and Monica lost her grandmother at the age of two. We lived next door to Mom, and we found her that dreadful morning.

Sitting in the phone booth that day, I realized that I could have done nothing to save my mother. I also realized that what had happened to her wasn't the same for Monica. She was alive and breathing and there were things I could do. I heard a voice say, "Leave no stone unturned." I reached for my notebook and made a list of my friends. I planned to call each of them and ask them to share my mission of saving Monica. I was rekindled with purpose and drive.

I left the safety of the phone booth and went back to Monica's room. With a deep breath, I pushed the door open. I repeated silently to myself, "We are okay right now!"

My friends were compassionate and anxious to help! Barb suggested harvesting the umbilical cord blood after my sister-in-law delivered her baby that month in case a bone marrow transplant was an option. My brother and his wife agreed with that suggestion!

My dear friend Pat suggested Reiki, which she happily did for Monica. Jill, another co-worker, shared a special closeness with Monica, and they called themselves "The Moth Sisters." Jill visited Monica in the hospital, providing lightness and laughter while also giving me a break. Other friends sent healing passages, healer's quotes, and holy water. They sent pendants, prayers, and affirmations or offered mantras, guided meditations, reflexology, and pressure point massages. Still others held fundraisers and blood drives.

The weeks turned into months. Some days, Monica was so sick she was transferred to the ICU. Then a miracle would happen, she would turn for the better, and be released from the ICU back to the children's cancer wing. The whole time, we did our best to stay in the moment.

Eventually the study concluded and, ten months after being admitted, she was released to go home. Her cancer was in remission!

I arranged for physical therapy to build Monica's strength up before she went back to school. Without missing a beat, she returned to school and picked up her friendships. No hair? no problem! Her friends wore hats or shaved their heads to help her fit in. And just like that, Monica was back in her world.

Me, not so much. I sat in the car thinking, *now what?* The experiences I had had over the year changed who I was. For eleven years I had been a busy real estate broker and appraiser with my own business. But I'd abandoned my work the day Monica was admitted to the hospital. I no longer felt that I could simply return to business as usual. Life had gone on just fine without me. I could no longer participate in small talk or listen to long stories about someone's annoyances. I felt in the wake of Monica's illness a sense that no one understood me. I lived in anticipation of her next follow-up visit to see if the leukemia was back. I couldn't be bothered by the trivial and shallow things of everyday life. I wanted to shout, "Children are dying of cancer today!" While at the same time I didn't want to shout it all; because I truly didn't want anyone else to feel the pain I felt.

Twenty-one years have passed, and as I write this, I reflect on the profound coincidences that often happened. And how I came to rely on both Monica's and my own instincts in order to ask questions and dig deeper. To recall the wonder of how, just the right thing or person showed up exactly when we needed it. Or how Monica miraculously recovered when I was told that she would pass within hours, not once, not twice, but seven times. There were enough miracles and coincidences to fill a book! Her primary oncologist went on to do his doctorate in natural medicine as her case truly made an impact on how he looked at alternatives to save patients. Monica's nurses stay in touch with us still to this day through social media as Monica is a constant reminder of hope and the possibility of experiencing miracles.

Monica and I solidly believed from the beginning that she would live. Through most of her treatments, that belief was all we had. We had no evidence, no statistics, no one convincing us to hang in there. Actually, we had the opposite—medical professionals who told us to have psychological interventions to help us accept her death and transition, as they considered it to be the certain outcome of her condition. The more they pushed for acceptance, the louder my inner voice grew—it was not Monica's time to die.

Once we were on the other side, I decided to take advantage of the pause. I followed my inner voice, and my heart because they were what I could hear. I couldn't explain why Monica had survived other than because we kept faith in her recovery. I didn't re-enter the bustle and demanding chaos of the real estate world that I had left behind. Instead, my interest in holistic health and healing alternatives claimed my focus.

I realized at the same time that my spirit became completely willing to let go of the only way I knew how to make a living. I am okay with that. Monica is alive. Truly that is all I asked for, so I am good. I vow to follow my inner guidance from this day forward, with full trust and faith, knowing that we are okay now.

Reflection

What events in your life have made you stop and look at everything differently?

_____

_____

_____

_____

What coincidences have you experienced that gave you evidence of the powerful universe beyond what we can see?

_____

_____

_____

_____

How has your "knowing" compelled you to move forward when the evidence was not there?

_____

_____

_____

_____

Learning to Be

VERONICA COLE

A doer life presents unending opportunities to *do*. There was only one thing I could not do: mend a broken spirit and a broken heart.

I loved Brooklyn in November! Leaves crunched underfoot, and the brisk autumn air smelled familiarly of home. I saw the row of red brick houses on the avenue, a well-worn path to my Canarsie neighborhood. *Soon, Veronica, soon.* My pace quickened as I wondered what dishes we'd prepare for our Thanksgiving feast. Perhaps we'd try a new recipe I'd discovered in *Bon Appetit.* In my mind, I visualized my mother inside my home, her perfectly coiffed hair and meticulous style, a true Leo. She was a *doer* like me. She could fix anything and always had the right words and comforting tone that only she possessed.

My key slid in the front door lock, and I smiled at the familiar *click* letting me in.

I bolted up three flights. "I'm home!"

My husband Charles stood just inside the door.

"Where's Mom?" I laid down my purse. My husband's gentle touch guided me into the bedroom.

My mother and sister Angela sat on the edge of our bed, crying softly. Not exactly the welcome I'd expected.

Charles's said, tenderly, "Christopher is dead."

Nooooo! My body dropped and folded, accordion-style. Christopher, the youngest of my five brothers, was only twenty. He and I were connected on a mercurial and heart level. He got me, my metaphysical views and devotion to the arts. I got him and his love of music as he claimed, Elvis was king.

How could he be dead? I could see his shock of blonde hair and six-foot frame. His laughter was quick and easy with a wit to match. He'd been found dead near our property, an unsolved mystery to this day.

I disassociated from my body, and I began to scream hysterically. Charles said something to me but I couldn't comprehend him. My body vibrated with disbelief. Everything appeared blurry, ghost-like, and unreal. Nobody mattered because I felt as though I had been ripped into tiny particles and thrown into space. I was everywhere and nowhere.

As a young child, I often became frightened with feelings and visions of my family members dying. These syncopated thoughts ended up with a warm hug and words of reassurance from my all-knowing mother. I wished my long-standing fear had been a wildly concocted child's dream.

I plodded along those early days after Christopher's death. Periodically, I would disappear into the pink-tiled ladies-room at the Manhattan office building where I worked, offering quick prayers that breathed life into me. I felt loved by the energy of spirit.

Metaphysics spoke to me, and my studies within that area gave me tools to actively invoke Spirit. I grew up Catholic, and it was from those day that my reverence for Spirit stemmed. Later, I chose to expand my beliefs. I appreciated the pomp and circumstance and incense of the Catholic faith but left the dogma behind.

I had been a full-time student at the American Academy of Dramatic Arts studying acting. After Christopher's death, getting out of bed was considered a triumph. I wondered what it was all for. Thankfully, my spiritual beliefs supported me. My foundation was built on something greater than me.

On a bright New York City morning, I rode the Command Bus from Brooklyn to Fifth Avenue. In a state halfway between sleeping and being awake, I had a sudden vision of my oldest brother Billy. I shook it off. When the bus reached Fifth Avenue, I jumped off and walked to the bank where I worked.

Just as I started my tasks, a phone call for me came into the switchboard. At my "hello," all I heard was, "Billy died." Billy had been on a trip to Georgia. To avoid an illegally parked truck on the rainy highway, he swerved, lost control of his truck, and slammed into a tree. He was killed instantly. Christopher had only been gone three months.

God, metaphysical thinking, and spiritual beliefs be damned. I was filled with inconsolable feelings of loss. On the plane ride to Billy's funeral, I curled into a ball, my face pressed against the window, and sobbed. Sorrow blended with fury. Faces of well-meaning family and friends swirled in my head. "This will never happen again. You have other brothers, right?" The mere sound of laughter brought up an impulse in me to scream. I was broken.

Billy had been solid in his devotion to me. After leaving for work, he would come to my place. As the doorbell rang, and I knew it was him because he was so consistent and reliable. He would plunk himself down on the wood stool in my kitchen and check in with me. I felt safe with him nearby. He made himself known and available—I had different kinds of affection from Christopher and Billy, who was always first to lend a hand. Death took those two pieces of my heart. I couldn't imagine enduring and recovering from those sudden losses.

With two of my brothers' sudden deaths, my beliefs no longer sustained me. My therapist Mary conveyed compassion with her calming voice and held space for the voluminous amounts of pain I presented to her. One day, as she sat in her maroon leather chair, pen poised over her notebook, she quietly told me, almost in a whisper, about the gifts she believed I possessed. Mary's keen intuition always amazed me. She suggested I investigate studying at The Institute for Modern Psychoanalysis. "You have a gift which can't be learned from a book. I think this may fill in the Swiss cheese holes for you concerning your brothers."

My zest for pursuing auditions, vocal lessons, and a desire to be in theatre dissipated. Those activities seemed frivolous in the wake of my brothers' deaths. I listened to Mary and checked out the institute.

The institute was a menagerie of students and professors who believed in the world of feelings and how releasing these feelings could provide healing. I found an emotional home which honored me for what I brought to the institute but also the brilliance in others. Slowly, I began to find a new path in my existence. The trajectory of my life changed in this experience. I knew I was where I was meant to be.

I became a holistic psychoanalytic psychotherapist and am deeply grateful for finding myself amongst the rubble. Pieces of me were reconstructed into a stronger, wiser, and more deeply compassionate human. I am now whole.

I am more than a *doer*. I can now BE.

Reflection

In what ways do you show up as a *doer* in your life? Are there opportunities to invite *being* instead?

_____

_____

_____

_____

How has loss changed the trajectory of your life?

_____

_____

_____

_____

What will it feel like to release any grief that is lodged in your body?

_____

_____

_____

_____

Coming Home to Myself

CATHY MCPHERSON

"Cathy, have you made any friends?" my best friend gently probed.

"Hey, Shona…I gotta go," I abruptly answered, cutting her off. I felt that familiar tightening in my throat and stopped myself from giving in to the stinging tears welling up behind my eyes.

Friendships! I'd struggled my whole life making friends and being asked about it brought up painful wounds I had worked so hard to hide. I had come by my walls honestly. I had needed them to survive—to keep me safe.

But how could I tell anyone the truth of how excruciatingly lonely I was, and that I had made a big mistake selling my home and moving to Italy?

Triggered, I grabbed my keys and was about to leave my apartment, when my eyes caught the words of the poem I had brought with me…words I didn't fully understand and yet they seemed to pull me so powerfully. Folding up the piece of paper, I stuffed it in the front pocket of my jeans.

I knew exactly where I was headed; it had become my sacred place. Walking quickly, I navigated my way through the streets and up the seemingly endless stairs to the San Miniato Cemetery.

Curling up on a secluded bench, the sun bright and warm on my face, I became aware of the stillness around me. Then, closing my eyes, I allowed the tears to spill down my face, unable to hold them in anymore.

My story began in Florence, Italy, "living the dream" and failing miserably. My divorce had just settled after a toxic eleven-year legal battle and I had arrived in Florence with beautiful dreams of exploring, shopping, taking photos, and truthfully, just being able to rest my exhausted body and soul.

No matter where we live, we still bring ourselves; with all of our insecurities, feelings of unworthiness…the parts of us that are yet to be healed. And my loving best friend, had just picked the scab off a wound that never seemed to heal.

Wiping the tears from my eyes, I reached into my pocket and pulled out the poem that called to my unhealed heart; the poem that had perhaps brought me all the way here to the other side of the world, so far away from all of the ways I had stayed hidden. I unfolded the paper, yearning to see its truth. It was a simple poem about coming home and I had spent a lifetime looking for "home" in others; clinging as though I was drowning, only to find myself painfully abandoned and rejected. But this poem was suggesting that home was *inside* of me. *That I could be my own place of refuge.* I took in a deep breath and let it out slowly. "Help me," I whispered.

There are times when I feel this *knowingness*—by the stillness in my soul—to let go and trust. And in that moment, I felt it.

Growing up in a physically and spiritually abusive home, my sister Wendy and I, had always shared everything…a bedroom, our clothes, and our dreams. Just one year older than me, *she* was my sense of home. We were "the girls." She was the leader who I devotedly followed, so longing to be just like her that I could not see who *I* was.

And then, at eighteen, Wendy got a little rash over the bridge of her nose, and a few spots on her arms. The doctors called it lupus and sent her home with some pills. But the spots were on the move, and before we knew it, they had gone down her throat, and spread over her entire body. She wasn't able to eat. Her hair started to fall out in clumps. Mom and Dad moved her from our bedroom to the living room couch. And in that one small move, I felt like I'd lost her. It was as if someone lifted the anchor from my life, and I felt lost and angry. For the first time in my life, I was alone.

On a freezing windy night in March, in the hospital where both Wendy and I had been born, my mom held one of Wendy's hands and I held the other.

Mom said, "She's leaving now," and with my heart completely breaking, I stroked her face and whispered over and over again how much I loved her. I understood that she needed to go. And then she left. Quietly. Softly. She was only twenty-seven.

I had lost my home.

I met him on the stormiest of nights with the rain coming down in sheets and lightning exploding in the sky. It was a year after Wendy died, and a friend had set us up to meet. He was so charming, and I was so hungry to be loved, to belong, to have my own safe home. I jumped into the relationship and held on, turning a blind eye to that familiar sick feeling in my stomach. And somewhere in that eleven-year marriage, all of my childhood dreams of being someone's chosen, cherished wife were destroyed, and I became a chameleon, *what color do you want me to be, and I'll change for you?* By the time I left him, I felt as though shame filled every cell of my body. *If only I had been pretty enough, thin enough or smart enough* ran endlessly through my mind. I just wanted to hide myself away, find a healing book, and re-emerge into the world only when I could finally lift my head up again.

I believe my life reimagined began while I was struggling through the mud of my life, while the tears poured down my face, when I had no more answers, my palms outstretched, surrendering all. I believe healing answers were already on the way, when on my knees, in desperation I cried out, only to be met with silence, believing that no-one was listening.

I now understand that it took leaving my home, to help me *come home.* I had only ever known how to be a daughter, the other half of "the girls," a wife, a mother, but I had had no idea who *I* really was. I had done so much healing work on these different aspects of my life…but now before me was an invitation for me to have the *willingness* to open myself to others, to begin to let down my walls of protection and be seen—to understand that I would be safe. I would be okay.

It was time to begin to write a new story.

Here's what I've learned to be true about pivotal moments. Sometimes they come softly. Gently. A few words strung together from a poem; an answer from a heart's cry that comes before you even know how to put it into words. An unfolding of events that, on hindsight, blows you away, even though in the moment it is happening, you have no idea that a transformation has even begun. Sometimes what is unfolding is beyond anything you could have imagined!

Day-by-day, people started to cross my path, often just while I was out walking my dogs on those narrow Florentine streets. Sometimes the path to healing is so simple. One beautiful soul asked if she could live with me, and I realized that in my *willingness* to be open, I was being asked not only to open my heart, but also my home. I said yes!

A community formed…one in which I felt valued and loved. I began to see myself, my colors, my worth, reflected back to me through their eyes. I was learning to be vulnerable, and I gently began to release my wounds, fears, and insecurities, finding within me that safe sanctuary I had longed for. *I was coming home to myself.*

On the other side of the darkness, there's so much beauty. I've learned to tell my story with compassion. Bringing into the light all the things I would normally keep hidden has allowed me to embrace all of me, giving me the ability to write a new today and tomorrow story. My healing journey will always continue to unfold…with my sister Wendy cheering me on from the other side!

With gratitude and joy, I have stepped fully into my life's purpose, walking side-by-side with women healing from trauma, abuse, and betrayal; sharing with them the healing tools that I have been given, as each one begins to find their own beauty with love and compassion, on their journey—the journey back home to themselves.

Reflection

What unhealed parts of your story would you simply be *willing* to allow your guides to help you heal? Can you list them and release them?

_____

_____

_____

_____

What are some of the ways that you are uniquely YOU that you may have struggled with in the past and can now appreciate and embrace? Where do you want to give yourself compassion?

_____

_____

_____

_____

Who are the people in your community that reflect the beautiful truth of who you are? What are the ways that you are able to give that gift back to others who cross your path?

101

_____

_____

_____

A Note from the Editor

DEBORAH KEVIN

*W*hen Linda Joy first approached me about stepping into the chief editor role for the *Life Reimagined* anthology, we hadn't yet heard of COVID-19 or imagined how quickly our collective lives would be reimagined, and on a global scale. Linda and I discussed how our own lives had been reimagined over the years, the sliding door moments, and divine timing of changes that brought us growth and joy. It was through this lens that we landed on the title, never imagining how perfectly-timed this anthology would be. Isn't the Universe amazing like that?

As their editor, I have had the privilege of reading first drafts of the courageous women who submitted their stories for inclusion in *Life Reimagined*—and their tales ranged from heartbreak over sudden loss, dissolution of marriages, honoring of life markers, and connecting with the Universe in new ways. As we worked through their revisions, I observed them standing a little taller, owning more of their badassery, and claiming themselves in new ways. That's one of the many gifts that came through the process of bringing *Life Reimagined* to publication.

My own life shifted in major ways at this time, too. During the quiet of the pandemic shut down, I had time to think and reflect: what was important to me and how would I leverage this new world reality to reimagine my life? I pursued a year-long master's degree in publishing and redefined how my Highlander Press publishing house would operate.

In August 2020, I suddenly lost my father and found myself grieving along with the rest of the world over the staggering loss of life. On the day of my dad's funeral, I asked for a sign from him—three butterflies—that he was well and happy in his new form. In his wisdom, my dad knew I would rationalize away three butterflies, so he sent *hundreds* of butterflies to three friends, none of whom knew I had asked for this sign or who lived anywhere near each other (one in Florida, one in Toronto, and the other in the United

Kingdom). I felt more connected to him than ever, and incredibly grateful for this continued communion. Thank you, Universe!

Then, during a guided meditation practice led by a dear friend of mine, I received a message that I was to reach out to the love of my life with whom I hadn't been in contact with for thirty years. My intention was to release his hold on my heart, bless him, and express my gratitude for who he had been in my life. Unbeknownst to me, he too harbored deep love and gratitude for me. I couldn't have imagined that we'd reconnect and begin reimagining our lives in a new way, full of ease, grace, and laughter. Once again, the Universe delivered!

My stories aren't unique—the women within these pages also shared similar experiences. The Universe always delivers the right people and projects into our lives at exactly the right time. The magic of it all continues to take my breath away.

As you dig into the stories of reimagined lives between these covers, I hope you too find Universal deliveries that shift your perspective, grow your heart, and allow you to step more fully into your badassery. And so it is.

With love and gratitude,

Deborah Kevin
Chief Editor, Inspired Living Publishing, LLC

ABOUT OUR
Authors

Christin Bjergbakke is The Usher Channeler, Reiki Master Teacher, and a past-life therapist, who guides her international clientele of women on how to stay centered in the heart and merge their soulful essence to life on Earth by unlocking the wisdom they carry within. She has published her first channeled book, and offers online coaching, including direct channeling from ascended masters, as well as live retreats. You can work with Christin in single sessions or monthly programs dedicated to your needs. Learn more at **www.usherchanneler.com**.

Sarah Breen is an Integrative Shamanic Energy Medicine Practitioner, author, and mentor. Her commitment is to cultivate sacred space helping those express their TRUE selves, living free of the chains of their ancestors' unexpressed lives. She supports her clients in writing a new map, one that is open to curiosity and awakening the wisdom that has never left. Embodying healing is the journey to becoming one with our light and dark. Learn more at **www.MindSpiritMapping.com**.

Kim Brochu, a personal empowerment coach, guides mindful women on their journey of self-love so they can heal their inner wounds, release limiting beliefs, and emerge as their most authentic selves. From that place of healing, they are empowered to become aligned with new beliefs so they can consciously create the life they desire. Kim customizes each client's experience, based on their inner wounds, by merging her intuitive abilities with her practical and spiritual tools. Learn more at **www.kimbrochu.com**.

As a Neuro-Transformational Coach™ **Cathy Casteel** is passionate about supporting and empowering highly sensitive empathic women, to release their layers of false beliefs so they can find their voice, reclaim their self-worth and begin living the authentic joy-filled life they desire. Cathy intuitively incorporates numerous methodologies to dive deep into a client's beliefs, values, emotions, drivers, and embodied traumas, allowing long lasting breakthroughs to sift into their lives, instead of constantly repeating the same self-sabotaging patterns. Learn more at **www.Cathy-Casteel.com**.

Cara Hope Clark, author of *Widow's Moon: A Memoir of Healing, Hope, and Self-Discovery Through Grief and Loss*, shares inspirational wisdom and assists others along their own journey through grief. She has been on a divinely guided path of personal and spiritual growth for over forty years. A former massage therapist and intuitive energy healer, her life purpose continues to be a guiding light for others. Learn more at: **www.carahopeclark.com**.

Crystal Cockerham is a spiritual mentor, certified Red Tent facilitator, international bestselling author, and the founder of Wisdom Awakens, LLC. She works with awakened, empathic women to unlock the shackles of pain, shame, and self-condemnation so they can reclaim their sovereignty and liberate themselves from the world's perceptions. Crystal works with women in private one-on-one sessions, group programs and spiritual retreats. Learn more at **www.CrystalCockerham.com**.

Veronica Cole is a licensed holistic psychotherapist, certified body-mind psychology coach, and certified grief specialist. Additionally, she's a certified Kundalini yoga instructor with a specialty in anxiety, depression and healing the inner child. She travels, works, and lives internationally, which expands her awareness of global diversity, spiritual beliefs, and practices. She has an extensive background working internationally with the military addressing issues of PTSD and combat related stress. She resides in Saratoga Springs, NY, with her husband, daughter, and beloved Maltese. Learn more at **www. facebook.com/veronicacole.adultsiblingloss**.

Robin Eaton is a spiritual teacher, shaman, and coach. She was initiated in the Q'ero traditions and lineage, is a Reiki Master Instructor, and a Master Neuro-Transformational™ Coach. Robin helps women dispel doubt and uncertainty to live unapologetically and abundantly in the truth of their being, aligned with their soul's calling and core values. She is on a mission to connect every woman with the voice and freedom of her soul. Learn more at **www.soultouchedbyrobin.com**.

Kelley Grimes, MSW, is a counselor, speaker, international bestselling author, *Aspire Magazine* expert columnist, and self-nurturing expert. She is passionate about empowering overwhelmed and exhausted individuals to live with more peace, joy, and meaning through the practice of self-nurturing. Kelley also provides professional and leadership development to organizations dedicated to making the world a better place. She is married to a board game maker, has two empowered daughters, and loves singing with a small women's group. Her book *The Art of Self-Nurturing: A Field Guide to Living With More Peace, Joy, and Meaning* was published in September 2020. Learn more at **www.cultivatingpeaceandjoy.com**.

Kris Groth, an Archangel life coach, intuitive energy healer, and sound healer, is the bestselling author of *Soul-iloquy: A Novel of Healing, Soul Connection & Passion*. Kris and her angels help women heal their hearts, nourish their souls, and illuminate their paths; empowering them to elevate higher and live their light! Kris serves clients around the world through healing and coaching sessions, online courses, and powerful guided sound healing meditations using crystal singing bowls. Learn more at **www.KrisGroth.com**.

From the time **Jami Hearn** was a child, she wanted to be a lawyer—she thought that was the path to a successful life. She built a successful law practice but remained unfulfilled…something more was calling her. Jami began to understand that what she did was not who she was. She embarked on a journey to create a thriving international consulting business helping women create the lives of their dreams without guilt, judgment or struggle. Learn more at **www.JamiHearn.com**.

Amber Kasic, a global citizen and lifelong learner, believes we all are spiritual beings capable of accessing our soul's personal and collective truths. While in her practical day-to-day life she is an award-winning educator and school partner dedicated to transforming teaching and learning through meaningful partnership, she also shares her transformational journey as a spiritual seeker and developing medium. To be inspired and connect with self, soul, or spirit, visit **www.natureswayopen.com**.

Donna LaBar, a certified Intuitive Health Coach, Emotion Code practitioner, and speaker, skillfully transforms her clients' health by integrating education with simple changes in daily habits, balancing their emotions, and moving away from past conditioning to build solid connections with their intuition and inner guidance. Donna's is recognized for the profound health restoration and fresh new direction enjoyed by her clientele. Her book, *Simple. Natural. Healing. A Commonsense Approach to Total Health Transformation*, is a must read. **www.donnalabar.com**.

Lisa Manyon is the business marketing architect and president of Write On Creative®. She pioneered the values-based Challenge. Solution. Invitation™ communication framework, to create marketing messages with integrity focusing on PASSION points. Her strategies are known to create million-dollar results. She's a cancer thriver who believes in healing with L♥VE. She shares her personal story, journal prompts, and inspiration, to help you heal yourself with love and redefine your relationship with self, health, and wealth via Spiritual Sugar™. Learn more at **www.SpiritualSugar.com**.

Cathy McPherson loves traveling, photography, and the grace of self-compassion. She is an NLP master practitioner and trained grief facilitator based in Ontario, Canada. Creator of the course, Becoming Whole: a nine-week journey back home to yourself, Cathy is passionate about walking side-by-side with women as they heal from trauma, loss, and betrayal. She guides them in healing their yesterday stories, empowering them to be the authentic creator of their today and tomorrow stories! Learn more at **www.findingyourbeauty.ca/becomingwhole**.

Nancy OKeefe, a certified Human Design Specialist, intuitive coach, and compassionate transformer, helps women peel back the layers of who they have been taught to be to reveal who they truly are so they can live their inner truth, go after their deepest desires, and create a life filled with success, satisfaction, and joy. Nancy has helped people bring out their best qualities for over twenty-five years. She can be found at **www.NancyOKeefeCoaching. com**.

Consciously merging her practical tools as a psychologist, in practice for over two decades, with her intuitive and spiritual gifts, Intuitive Psychologist **Dr. Debra Reble** empowers women to connect with their hearts, release fear and anxiety, and supports them in breaking through their energetic and spiritual blocks to self-love so they can live authentically. Debra is a sought-after speaker and media guest and is the host of the popular Soul-Hearted Living podcast on iTunes. She can be found at **www.debrareble.com**.

Angela Shakti Sparks is a holistic wellness coach, certified crystal practitioner, hypnotherapist, Neurolinguistic Programming (NLP) master practitioner, and founder of Evolved Energetics energy healing. She combines proven methods from these disciplines that create deep and lasting change rapidly. She specializes in working with empaths, highly sensitive people (HSPs), and women with anxiety, depression, and chronic health conditions. Learn more: **www.angelashaktisparks.com**.

Dr. Lisa Thompson, an Intuitive Transformational Coach, empowers women to intentionally design their best life by living from "yes," so they can embrace self-love, trust their intuition, and gracefully move forward through their fears to take inspired action to live a life they love. She is the bestselling author of *Sacred Soul Love* and *Sacred Soul Spaces*. She leads destination retreats and teaches online courses. For more information, visit **www.DrLisaJThompson. com**.

Kimmberly Wotipka is passionate about helping women tap into their inner radiant queens, enabling them to harness their spiritual power, manifest their deepest desires, and create radiant lives. A certified Emotional Freedom Technique (EFT) practitioner with degrees in business and spiritual studies, she's an entrepreneur with a big heart. Kimmberly is honored to help women live a life that makes them feel like royalty every single day. Learn more at **www.TheRadiantQueen.com**.

ABOUT OUR
Publisher

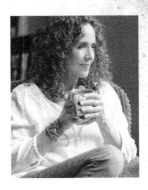

$\mathcal{F}$ounded in 2010 by Sacred Visibility™ Catalyst, Intentional Living Guide,™ Mindset Mojo Mentor,™ radio show host, and Aspire Magazine Publisher Linda Joy, Inspired Living Publishing, LLC (ILP), is a bestselling boutique hybrid publishing company.

Dedicated to publishing books for women and by women and to spreading a message of love, positivity, feminine wisdom, and self-empowerment to women of all ages, backgrounds, and life paths—Inspired Living Publishing's books have reached numerous international bestseller lists as well as Amazon's Movers & Shakers lists.

The company's authors benefit from Linda's family of multimedia inspirational brands that reach over 44,000 subscribers and a thriving social media community.

Inspired Living Publishing works with mission-driven, heart-centered female entrepreneurs—life, business, and spiritual coaches, therapists, service providers, and health practitioners in the personal and spiritual development genres, to bring their message and mission to life and to the world. ILP publishes, markets and launches select manuscripts by transformational female authors whose messages are aligned with their philosophy of inspiration, authenticity, empowerment, and personal transformation.

Through Inspired Living Publishing's highly successful sacred anthology division, hundreds of visionary female entrepreneurs have written their sacred soul stories using ILP's Authentic Storytelling™ writing model and became bestselling authors.

What sets Inspired Living Publishing™ apart is the powerful, high-visibility publishing, marketing, bestseller launch, and exposure across multiple media platforms that are included in its publishing packages. Their family of authors reap the benefits of being a part of a sacred family of inspirational multimedia brands that deliver the best in transformational and empowering content across a wide range of platforms—and has been doing so since 2006 with the birth of Aspire Magazine.

Linda also works privately with empowered female entrepreneurs and messengers through her Illuminate Sistermind™ Program and other visibility-enhancing offerings. Linda's other visibility-enhancing brands including Inspired Living Secrets™, Inspired Living Giveaway™, Inspired Living University™, and her popular radio show, Inspired Conversations. Learn more about Linda's private work and offerings at www.Linda-Joy.com.

If you're ready to publish your transformational book or share your story in one of ours, we invite you to join us! Learn more about our publishing services at **InspiredLivingPublishing.com.**

Inspired Living Publishing ~ Transforming Women's Lives, One Story at a Time™

If you enjoyed this book, visit
www.InspiredLivingPublishing.com
and sign up for ILP's e-zine to receive news about hot new releases, promotions, and information on exciting author events.

ABOUT OUR
Editor

DEBORAH KEVIN

*W*riter, editor, and storyteller Deborah Kevin, chief inspiration officer of Highlander Press, is the chief editor for Inspired Living Publishing and a former editor of *Little Patuxent Review*.

Deborah's editorial portfolio includes ILP's *Shine!*, *Courageous Hearts*, *The Art of Self-Nurturing*, and *Soul-Hearted Living*. Her essays and interviews have been published by *Aspire Magazine*, *Equitas International*, Karen Salmansohn, *Little Patuxent Review*, and *166 Palms*.

A graduate of Stanford University's novel writing program, Deborah also earned a master's degree in publishing from Western Colorado University. Her first novel, *Finding Grace*, is slated for publication in 2022.

Deborah splits her time between a city home in Baltimore, Maryland, and a country home in New Jersey, with the love of her life, Rob, two sons, and their pups, Fergus and Nikko. When she's not writing or editing, Deborah can be found hiking, kayaking, dancing, cooking, and traveling. Learn more about Deborah's work at DeborahKevin.com.

Made in the USA
Coppell, TX
09 November 2021

65477257R00077